Praise for █

"This is an important book. *Closure* highlights the social and professional harm caused by decisions made in secret with bad data. The lack of transparency, the dissembling and the vindictiveness is here in all its ugly predictability. I hope this is not the end of the story."
Nick Wallis, author of *The Great Post Office Scandal*

"We have long known that there is a significant problem in the maternity services, and it's not the one that you read about in the press. The real problem is the systematic devaluing and disintegration of models of care that follow the evidence, support female physiology, and promote autonomous midwifery practice. This book is important because it doesn't just tell us *that* this happens: it shows us *how* it happened to one group of midwives and the women and families they were caring for. I desperately wish that *Closure* had never needed to be written, but it is really important that it has been. We have much to learn from it."
Dr Sara Wickham, author and researcher

"The Albany Midwifery Practice informed the development of best practice midwifery care in many countries, including Australia. Midwives and policy leaders drew substantially from both the theory underpinning the practice as well as the design and implementation aspects that delivered such excellent outcomes. This is a page-turning story of how an exemplary, internationally acclaimed service was closed down. It acts as a warning about how complex power dynamics within contemporary maternity care can threaten and undermine the development of services that lead to positive experiences for women and families."
Pat Brodie, Professor of Midwifery, Member of the Order of Australia

"This book is a crucial part of the story of midwifery: it absolutely needs to be widely read."
Gill Boden, psychologist and birth activist working with asylum seekers

"A fascinating, well-constructed and easily readable account of misguided damage to a gold standard maternity care service. The story illustrates many of the ways in which poor quality and lack of good leadership, and lack of accountability continues to imperil good health care, and fails staff and patients."
Andy Beckingham, Consultant in Public Health

"The Albany Midwifery Practice was an inspired innovation. It put women at the heart of everything and it gave mothers a voice that was louder than any profession. This story is evocative of what has happened to so many exceptional midwifery pilots, projects and innovations. Why are midwives so threatening when they succeed with services that give women what they ask for? I believe the answers are in this book. Every midwife in the UK should read this story. It is heart-wrenching in its truth, and you will shed tears for the women who have been left without the promise of midwife-mother relationships. The power of midwives and women working together is invincible. The outcomes of the Albany Practice were what any modern service should be aiming for."
Dr Kathryn Gutteridge, Midwife

"*Closure* describes one of the biggest tragedies the birth world has ever seen. The Albany midwives offered the care that most women want – care that is personalised, community-based and culturally safe. Failure to recognise this when determining safe maternity care is an injustice that will play out for decades to come, to the detriment of many. This book finally gives us an honest account of what led to the closure of such an exemplary midwifery practice. Each page of the book leaves you wanting to read more…"
Michelle Quashie, maternity improvement campaigner and founder of the Women's Voices Conference

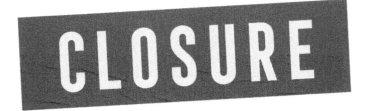

CLOSURE

How the flagship Albany
Midwifery Practice, at the heart
of its South London community,
was demonised and dismantled

Becky Reed & Nadine Edwards

pinter
&
martin

Closure: How the flagship Albany Midwifery Practice, at the heart of its South London community, was demonised and dismantled

First published by Pinter & Martin 2023

© 2023 Becky Reed and Nadine Edwards

The authors have asserted their moral rights to be identified as the author of this work in accordance with the Copyright, Designs and Patents Act of 1988.

ISBN 978-1-78066-785-0

Also available as ebook

British Library Cataloguing-in-Publication Data
A catalogue record for this book is available from the British Library.

Set in Dante

Printed and bound by Severn

Pinter & Martin Ltd
6 Effra Parade
London SW2 1PS

pinterandmartin.com

Contents

For all the midwives and others who worked
in the Albany Midwifery Practice 1997–2009

For all the women and families of Peckham
who trusted the midwives with their care

And in memory of Beverley Lawrence Beech
1944–2023

'In fear of difference, in fear of excellence.'
Mavis Kirkham

'The closing of the Albany practice will stand as a tragedy in childbirth history in which authoritarian misinformed leadership destroyed an almost perfect care model, depriving women who had depended on the Albany midwives for years of ongoing and highly effective care, placed dynamic midwifery careers on hold, and destroyed relationships that could instead have worked in unison for the better good. It will stand forever as an example of how not to base decisions on politics and inappropriate categorization of data. Let's hope its closing will be a model of misfortune not to be repeated.'
Betty-Anne Daviss

Foreword

The Albany Practice was probably the most researched and audited midwifery practice in the world. This is one of the reasons why the story of its closure by King's College Hospital is so important. The Practice's clinical and social outcomes were excellent. It gave midwives a level of job satisfaction rarely experienced in modern fragmented maternity services. It was loved by those receiving its services and by other midwives who aspired to work in a similar manner, as shown by the demonstrations after the closure. The process by which a practice with such a fine reputation came to be closed merits attention, if the sad state of NHS maternity services is to be improved. All those involved with maternity services can therefore learn from the tragic processes revealed in this book.

Becky Reed was an Albany midwife of long standing, who was witch-hunted as part of the closure processes (see Chapter 20). Nadine Edwards is a birth activist who was involved in the campaign to save the Albany, and whose writing and practical work have helped so many women. These two together are ideally placed to write this book. As a midwife researcher, I was impressed with the Albany Practice and encouraged those involved to write about how it worked.[1] I am therefore honoured to be asked to write this foreword, though greatly saddened that the events here described ever happened.

This book is also important for what it demonstrates about the culture of NHS maternity services. I believe 'Your workplace culture is defined by the worst thing you allow to happen in your workplace. That worst thing/activity/event defines your workplace.'[2] This book concerns the worst aspect of the culture of NHS maternity services and there is much to learn from this case study of its operation.

The story of the closure of the Albany Midwifery Practice

concerns the scything of tall poppies by those seeking to protect the status quo, even though the Albany Practice was achieving the aims of NHS maternity services by means which have been policy since the publication of *Changing Childbirth* in 1993.[3] Such defensive scything has a long history[4] and is seen in the closure of birth centres and projects where services are local and offer continuity of carer, though it is those very factors that improve outcomes for mothers and babies.

The closure also highlights a profound cultural clash between the technological imperative within the current industrial model of maternity care in the NHS and the relationship-based approach of continuity of midwifery care on which the Albany Practice was based. The industrial model, dominant in the NHS and in our society, sees birth as a mechanical process which needs to be tightly controlled for maximum efficiency. By this logic, the centralisation and standardisation of maternity services aids efficiency. The fragmentation of care, so as to address potential problems or risks, then follows. Such organisation of the service makes possible and necessary the management assumption that midwives provide specialised fragments of maternity care and can be moved to plug the gaps in the service, despite the negative impact on their morale. The technological imperative, honed in industry and fundamental to our economic system, requires the problems the service addresses to be defined in detail and assumes that only technology can solve them. One problem with such a standardised service is that it treats all childbearing women as the same. Another problem is that it does not address their social context.

The relationship model, on which midwifery was long based, is built on the assumption that birth is fundamentally something that women do, and that women differ from one another. This model sees birth as grounded in relationships, and the mother's trust in herself and her carer is developed over time. Where the mother's relationship with a midwife she knows and trusts is at the centre of care, that care is adapted to suit the individual and her self-confidence and understanding grows, with profound and positive physiological and social results. The relationship with her midwife also develops in the context of the woman's life. For instance, antenatal education at the Albany Practice was offered through discussion in groups of pregnant and postnatal women with their midwives. This enabled women to learn from their peers as well as their midwives and go on to tell their own stories after their babies were born, thus developing confidence as well as relevant knowledge. These groups were also designed to enable women to develop in pregnancy the friendship networks which are so important for new mothers.[1]

One 'problem' with continuity of midwifery care is that as midwives' relationships develop with the women in their care, so does their loyalty to those mothers, which can be seen as lessening their loyalty to their employer.[5] The Albany midwives had foreseen this and negotiated a contract in which they remained self-employed. But this did not prevent their primary commitment to the women in their care being seen as threatening and subversive within the management structures of a hospital organised on a very different model. Or was it that the relative autonomy enjoyed by Albany mothers and midwives was seen as intolerable, despite its good outcomes?

If birth is grounded in relationships, whether sustained or fragmented, so too are maternity services and parallel processes become apparent. Where midwives are trusted, as Cathy Warwick, the Head of Midwifery at King's, trusted the Albany midwives, midwives can trust mothers and as they become strong and confident together clinical outcomes improve. Where midwives are tightly controlled, bullied and fearful, they go on to treat mothers as they themselves are treated: mothers become fearful and compliant, birth interventions increase, and midwives leave midwifery. The witch-hunt against Becky shows how this toxic culture of blame has permeated the whole bureaucracy of UK midwifery.

There is a great deal we can learn from the sad story of this book. If we can name the processes which unfold in this story when they reappear, it might be possible to identify the 'rumblings' which here preceded the scything, discuss them openly and prevent it happening again. When we understand that innovative projects at grassroots level, which may be policy but which are outside the prevailing culture, need a protector, then such a role can be identified and appropriately filled. This is true of profound innovation in many spheres, not just around birth.[6]

In the same year that the Albany was closed down, the Practice was featured in the 2009 book *Birth Models that Work*.[7] When we understand that the successful models of midwifery care described in the book, like the Albany Midwifery Practice, usually serve a local area with continuity of midwifery carer, and also include good management and obstetric support, we will be able to prevent the tragic situation in which they are systematically closed or threatened with closure.

The model currently running NHS maternity services is driven by the dominant economic system,[8] which could be seen as using only one side of the brain.[9] It has produced a culture of bullying, fear and witch-hunting among midwives. This is reflected in the experience of pregnant and birthing women, who so often report feeling trapped on a conveyor belt. The relational midwifery model and the technological obstetric model should be complementary parts of a whole service, with mutual respect flowing between them. The Albany model was designed to achieve this. Childbirth, which is such an intensely personal and creative process, is not well served by an industrial model. The current alliance of the industrial and medical models bolsters an arrogance which protects the centralisation of power, creating a culture which enforces conformity and prevents grass-roots innovation. At a time when limited funding is starving the NHS, a toxic culture within the service is highly destructive. Those involved have told their story here. We must learn from them before it is too late.

Mavis Kirkham
Professor of Midwifery Emerita,
Sheffield Hallam University, England

References

1. Leap, N. (2010) The less we do the more we give. In Kirkham, M. Ed, *The Midwife-Mother Relationship*. Second Edition, Basingstoke, Macmillan.

2. Margaret E. Ward, eminent Irish journalist, 'Sexism at Work' on RTE Radio 1, Jan 25 2022.

3. Department of Health (1993) *Changing Childbirth: Report of the Expert Maternity Group*. London, HMSO.

4. The scything of tall poppies is a concept from ancient Greece with accounts in Herodotus' *Histories* (Book 5, 2f), Aristotle's *Politics* (1284a), and Livy's *Ab Urbe Condita Libri*, Book I.

5. Brodie, P. (1996) 'Australian Team Midwives in Transition'. Oslo, International Confederation of Midwives, 23rd Triennial Conference.

6. Ibbott, R. (2014) *Ujamaa: The Hidden Story of Tanzania's Socialist Villages*. London, Crossroads Books.

7. Davis-Floyd, R., Barclay, L., Davies, B.A. and Tritten, J. (2009) *Birth Models that Work*. Berkeley, University of California Press.

8. Kirkham, M. (2017) 'A Fundamental Contradiction: the business model does not fit midwifery values'. *Midwifery Matters* 152, 13-15.

9. McGilchrist, I. (2009) *The Master and his Emissary*, New Haven, Yale University Press.

Introduction:
The untold story

During the years 1997–2009 the Albany Midwifery Practice in London became known nationally and internationally as a midwifery model that exemplified excellent maternity care, with outstanding health outcomes for both mothers and babies and satisfaction for women and families. It provided a rewarding way of working for midwives, which also increased their midwifery knowledge and skills. In 2009, it was closed down by the hospital Trust to which it was contracted. The Trust claimed that the closure was for 'safety reasons', but this book tells a very different story.

When the Albany Midwifery Practice was closed, Zoe, one of the midwives working in the Practice at the time, commented:

> 'It feels like we were never really able to tell our side of the story. That there was an official story that was told that wasn't ours, and that we didn't feel was the story.'

So our aim has always been to tell the 'untold story'. We have been consistently reminded about the importance of doing this. Dr Luke Zander, a retired general practitioner (GP) from London who has his own significant part in the narrative, felt strongly that the story of the closure needed to be told: 'From the outside, it was much too important to just let it go'.

However, in the years following the closure, and after the ensuing three and a half year investigation into her practice, Becky was nowhere near ready to embark on telling this shocking and harrowing tale. It was too recent, too raw, too emotional.

By 2015 the idea of an 'Albany book' was feeling more important than ever. Becky emailed Nadine Edwards, who had been pivotal in the campaigns following the closure, and who was still closely involved in the ongoing quest for justice, to ask her how she would feel about working on a book together. Nadine replied that she would be honoured to do this. Thus the happy collaboration that led to this book began.

Early on we decided to try and interview as many of those involved in the story as possible, and with two important exceptions (the Head of Midwifery at the time, Katie Yiannouzis, and the Albany midwives' link obstetrician, Leonie Penna) all those we approached were more than willing and gave generously of their time, memories and insights. We also had several large dossiers of documentation, containing records meticulously kept by the midwives in the Practice as the events in this book were taking place. These files and boxes were filled with many hundreds of letters, emails, official responses and documents, research papers, press articles and more. We therefore had a great deal of reliable material and many personal recollections to draw on.

The title of the book, *Closure*, describes exactly that: the summary closure of the world-renowned Albany Midwifery Practice after 12 and a half successful years. This title was chosen in recognition not just of the events the book describes, but also to acknowledge the importance of trying to bring some closure to all those involved.

Closure is an attempt to make sense of why the events leading up to and during the closure of the Albany Practice unfolded as they did, and to try and understand how a well-loved midwifery practice achieving excellent, internationally acclaimed outcomes could be seen in any other way. The book also describes the events in the years following the closure, when many people in the local community of Peckham and beyond devoted their time and energy to what turned into an extraordinary campaign. We hope that by exposing the injustices that were perpetrated in so many people's lives, the emotional trauma that they have suffered for so many years will be alleviated.

We would especially like to honour the midwives working in the Practice at the time, all of whom were deeply affected by what happened, and we hope that in telling their story we have done them the justice they deserve. We also pay tribute to all the remarkable women and families who were involved either at the time or during the ensuing 'Save the Albany' campaign.

The book is intended to be an accessible and engaging account of the events it describes, highlighting nonetheless some of the deeply complex and distressing political failures of our times. The Albany story sits within a context of a wide range of failing institutions, poor accountability within these institutions and a democratic deficit built into the fabric of publicly funded institutions supposedly set up to serve and protect the general population.

As in the recent shocking scandal involving post office workers unfairly accused of fraud,* the lack of response and accountability, and a wilful blindness to consider a different perspective, are all too common. In the case of the Albany, flawed statistics took precedence over years of excellent outcomes. And unsurprisingly the women's and midwives' positive experiences, and the passionate campaigning of the local community, counted for nothing.

We hope that the principles of solidarity, care and community support embedded in the Albany model will inspire and serve as an exemplar for what can be achieved in maternity services of the future, if the political will, leadership and funding is there to support it.

---

* See Nick Wallis (2021) *The Great Post Office Scandal: The fight to expose a multimillion pound IT disaster which put innocent people in jail*, Bath Publishing.

The Albany Midwifery Practice Model (1997-2009)

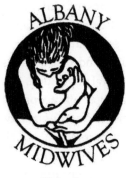

Albany logo

In 1994, following the 1993 government report *Changing Childbirth*, a group of midwives set up a new midwifery practice in Deptford in south-east London. The practice was known as the South East London Midwifery Group Practice (SELMGP), and ran very successfully, with excellent outcomes and growing popularity, until 1997, when the Health Authority funding that it relied on came to an end.

The practice was relocated to Peckham, a few miles away, and was renamed the Albany Midwifery Practice (AMP), with reference to the Albany Centre in Deptford where SELMGP had been situated, and in recognition of one of the local roads (Albany Road), which formed the boundary of its new 'patch'. The midwives successfully negotiated the first-ever contract with a National Health Service (NHS) Trust, and the AMP became the first group of NHS midwives working as a self-employed, self-managed practice, based in the community and offering continuity of carer to an individual caseload of women.

The AMP offered continuity of midwifery care with two midwives for each woman, known as a 'primary' and a 'second' midwife. These midwives provided antenatal and labour care, and postnatal care for up to 28 days (compared with the normal follow-up at the time of 10–14 days). Women were referred by local general practitioners (GPs), with occasional self-referrals, and some referrals from consultant obstetricians at King's College Hospital. The midwives looked after all the women regardless of their obstetric, medical, or social risk. Each 'whole caseload' midwife looked after 36 women a year as a primary midwife and a further

The Albany philosophy

- Pregnancy and birth are seen as a normal part of a woman's life.
- Midwifery care is a trusting, mutually respectful partnership between the woman and her carers.
- Each woman is entitled to get to know the midwives caring for her throughout her pregnancy and childbirth regardless of recognised risk factors, complications, or place of birth.
- Women should be able to give birth to their babies in a safe and satisfying way in the place of their choice.
- The midwife 'follows the woman', thereby enabling care either at home or in the hospital, as appropriate to the woman's needs and choices.
- Women have the right to be given evidence-based information in order to make informed choices throughout pregnancy, birth and the postnatal period.

36 as a second midwife, and the two 'half caseload' midwives looked after 18 'primaries' and 18 'seconds'. The midwives had 12 weeks' holiday a year, organised well in advance, and were on call for the women in their caseload at all times unless they were on holiday. The women knew that they could contact their midwives at any time if they needed to, but were asked not to call with non-urgent messages after 8pm or at weekends. The midwives arranged between themselves any special time off to attend important, unmissable social or family events. On average a midwife with a full caseload attended eight births a month, four as a primary and four as a second midwife.

Fundamental to the model were the two practice support workers. The practice administrator handled referrals and acted as general secretary for the midwives, while the manager dealt with media requests, organised workshops, and was the contact point for any national and international interest in the Practice.

As the referrals arrived, each woman was allocated a primary and a second midwife whose planned holidays didn't coincide with her estimated due date. The primary midwife was responsible for the woman's midwifery care and kept an overview of her individual situation. This midwife met the woman at home for a first (booking) visit, during which she took the woman's details and discussed her antenatal care, including referrals for any screening tests. Further antenatal visits were usually at the Practice at a time convenient for both the woman and her midwife. The second midwife also built up a relationship with the woman, sharing her antenatal care and always being part of the 'Birth Talk', a visit at around 36 weeks of pregnancy in the woman's home. This visit was seen as important preparation not only for the woman, but also for everyone planning to be involved in the birth.

The primary midwife arranged any necessary consultations with other professionals, and always accompanied women in her caseload to any obstetric appointments. The midwives worked very closely with their link obstetrician, keeping in contact regarding any women in their caseload who required obstetric input.

Choice of place of birth was discussed at the booking visit, and home birth was always presented positively, as the midwives knew that for a healthy woman this would increase her chance of having a straightforward birth.

Both the woman's named midwives planned to attend her birth, with the primary midwife calling the second when the birth was near or at any time she felt in need of support. The midwives carried their equipment with them at all times, and visited all women at home in labour, giving them the opportunity to make a final choice about place of birth at this time. In a long labour, the two midwives shared the care, and tried to ensure that the woman's primary midwife was with her when her baby was born. The primary midwife provided most of the postnatal care, with the second midwife usually doing one visit. The midwives were on call

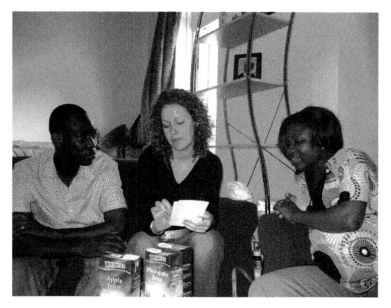

Danielle meeting Sade and her husband for a Birth Talk at home

for up to 28 days postnatally, and visited new mothers as needed during this time, encouraging them to start attending the postnatal group at the Practice when they felt ready.

Antenatal and postnatal groups were integral to the Albany model of care. The midwives facilitated three groups a week: an afternoon antenatal group for women only, an evening group where partners were welcome, and a postnatal group. All the pregnant women and new mothers were encouraged to attend, to share information and experiences, to learn from each other, and build supportive networks to help them as they became mothers.

Instead of always working in the same pairs, the midwives worked with different midwives in the group, which enabled them to develop and maintain a shared philosophy and approach, as well as learning from each other and being able to discuss births together.

Regular meetings were considered important in the Practice. At the start of each week, all the midwives and the practice manager

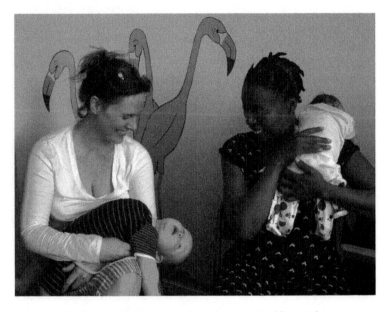

Mothers and babies at a postnatal group at Peckham Pulse

met to discuss any Practice business. During this meeting, they also had a 'how are we?' session, where they shared what had been happening and how they were feeling; this was seen to be very important because they were all working so closely together. The midwives also met over lunch once a week to share knowledge and discuss any interesting clinical issues.

In this model of care, known as 'relational continuity', each midwife is on call only for the women in her own caseload, ensuring that the women know their midwives and the midwives know the women who will be calling them. Thus a trusting, respectful relationship is built up between midwives and women, leading to improved satisfaction for mothers and families, as well as outstanding clinical outcomes for both mothers and babies.

Relational continuity of midwifery care supports all women, babies and families in the best possible way. In a trusting and continuous relationship women can talk about their past experiences and share openly any problems and fears. They can then move forward to a safe and satisfying birth experience, and a supportive start to motherhood.

Illustrating the importance to women of this model of care, an Albany mum, Farida, commented:

> *'Seeing the same person... you're not afraid. ...It's nice to see the same friendly face. You can also express your feelings more about any problems you may have. Just to know that you know who to contact, and you know who you're contacting at the same time.'*

The people in this story
(with their roles at the time)

Albany Midwifery Practice

Midwives

Mary Ardill

Fran Chambers

Danielle Clover

Natalie Doherty

Melissa Earle

Nicky Gibbs

Zoe Lench

Becky Reed

Zoe Vowles

Sophie Whitecross

Practice manager

Pauline Armstrong

King's College Hospital personnel

Kate Brintworth – Community Matron and Supervisor of
  Midwives

Tony Davies – Risk Management Obstetrician

Sarah Dawson – Divisional General Manager for Women and
  Children

Jill Demilew – Consultant Midwife and Supervisor of Midwives

Jacqueline Docherty – Deputy Chief Executive

Mike Marsh – AMP Link Obstetrician (2002–03)

Leonie Penna – AMP Link Obstetrician (2004–09)

Linda Sherratt – Risk Management Midwife

Roland Sinker – Director of Operations

Tim Smart – Chief Executive

Geraldine Walters – Director of Nursing and Midwifery

Cathy Walton – Consultant Midwife

Cathy Warwick – Former Director of Midwifery and General Manager, Women's and Children's Services (until 2008)

Katie Yiannouzis – Head of Midwifery and Supervisor of Midwives

Royal College of Midwives (RCM)

Francine Allen – Regional Officer

Pat Gould – Senior Representative in Becky Reed's Nursing and Midwifery Council (NMC) case

Carol King – Local Representative

Cathy Warwick – Chief Executive (2008–2017)

Midwifery Supervision

Angela Helleur – Local Supervising Authority Midwifery Officer, London

Jackie Moulla – Supervisor of Midwives

Nursing and Midwifery Council

Jackie Smith – Chief Executive

CEMACH/CMACE

Rachel Thomas – Senior Midwife, The London Project

Albany Campaign Members

The Albany midwives

Pauline Armstrong, member of Albany Action Group (AAG) and Albany Model Action Group (AMAG)

Emma Beamish – Founder of Albany Mums, member of AAG

Beverley Beech – Chair of the Association for Improvements in the Maternity Services (AIMS), member of AAG

Sarah Davies – Senior Midwifery Lecturer, University of Salford, member of AAG and AMAG

Nadine Edwards – Vice-chair of AIMS, member of AAG and AMAG

Caroline Flint – Former President of the Royal College of Midwives, member of AAG

Margaret Jowitt – Editor *Midwifery Matters* magazine, member of AAG

Mavis Kirkham – Professor of Midwifery Emerita, Sheffield
Hallam University, researcher and author, member of AAG
and AMAG

Jo Murphy-Lawless – sociologist and Midwifery Lecturer, Trinity
College Dublin, member of AAG and AMAG

Rix Pyke – Albany Mum, member of AAG, writer of campaign
songs

Wendy Savage – retired obstetrician, member of AAG

Luke Zander – retired GP, founder of Royal Society of Medicine's
Maternity and Newborn Forum, founder of AMAG

Statisticians

Jane Galbraith – Honorary Senior Research Associate in the
Department of Statistical Science, University College London

Alison Macfarlane – Professor of Perinatal Health, City University
London (now City, University of London)

Legal Support

Eleena Misra – barrister

Elizabeth Prochaska – human rights barrister, co-founder of
Birthrights charity

Politicians

Baroness Julia Cumberlege (House of Lords) – author of *Changing
Childbirth*

Norman Lamb, MP – Liberal Democrats Health Spokesman

Other Health Professionals

Mark Ashworth – GP, Peckham, London

Jane Sandall – Professor of Midwifery, King's College University,
London, researcher and author

Denis Walsh – Associate Professor of Midwifery, University of
Nottingham

1
Trouble brewing

Wednesday 3 December 2008

The phone rang. Becky was finishing her breakfast at home and thinking about organising her day's work. She was surprised to hear Leonie Penna's voice: Leonie was a friend of the Albany midwives and their named 'link obstetrician'. They consulted her when any woman they were looking after needed medical as well as midwifery support. But Leonie didn't ever ring the midwives at home. Her voice sounded serious. She was ringing to summon Becky to a meeting at the hospital that had already been arranged for later that morning. Attendance at the meeting was non-negotiable. Becky asked what the meeting was about and why she was being told to attend at such short notice, but Leonie refused to explain, repeating that attendance was obligatory.

Putting down the phone, Becky felt shocked and confused; she had no idea what such an apparently urgent meeting could possibly be about. She immediately phoned her midwife colleagues. It turned out that all six of them had just received a message on their pagers about attending the meeting, including those on annual leave. One of the midwives, Mary, described being called to the meeting as feeling like a 'three-line whip'. Another colleague, Nicky, found it 'overwhelming and scary'. No one had any idea why the meeting had been called without any warning, and everyone felt anxious and concerned.

What could it possibly be about? The idea of going to a meeting that sounded so serious was frankly terrifying. Without any knowledge of the agenda, the situation felt intimidating and unsafe. It was quickly decided that support was needed, and it was agreed that Mary would contact the local union representative, Carol, from the Royal College of Midwives. To the midwives' relief she was available, and agreed to come along for support and to take minutes of the meeting.

Mary, Danielle, Natalie, Nicky, Fran and Becky met Carol at King's College Hospital later that morning. As they all made their way to the meeting room, they felt a growing sense of foreboding. They were shown into a large room where the atmosphere felt hostile. They were faced with a group of five unsmiling senior doctors and midwives sitting on one side of a long rectangular table. These included the Head of Midwifery, Katie Yiannouzis, and Leonie Penna, the obstetrician who had phoned Becky earlier. Also present were Jean Yearwood, Community Midwifery Manager, Jill Demilew, Community Consultant Midwife, and Tony Davies, Consultant Obstetrician and Lead for Risk Management. The midwives were asked to sit down opposite them. The power imbalance in the room was almost tangible. It felt like an inquisition was about to begin.

Carol was introduced as a union representative and minute-taker for the midwives. There was no one taking minutes on the other side of the table. And then the accusations started: Leonie Penna, stabbing her finger across the table directly at Becky, began accusing the midwives of dangerous practice, saying 'you are responsible for 75% of all the admissions to special care of babies with HIE'. (HIE stands for hypoxic ischaemic encephalopathy, a form of brain damage.) She pushed a printed document, titled 'Term Babies Born in Very Poor Condition', across the table to the midwives. Natalie remembers the midwives 'all staring at those flimsy scraps of poorly presented data… [which] felt like something from a bad school project.'

This document, which turned out to be the first of three versions, would subsequently be referred to as the 'Case Series'. The figures on the front page looked as though they supported the claim about babies with HIE admitted to special care, apparently showing that of 16 babies admitted over 31 months and one day, 12 were Albany babies. The midwives couldn't believe what they were hearing, and Becky questioned where the figures had come from. The midwives were all in shock, and Mary was in tears.

It was obvious that a plan had already been made about what to do next. Katie Yiannouzis explained that those present were so concerned about the apparent damage to Albany babies that they had decided to act immediately. An external review by the Confidential Enquiry into Maternal and Child Health (CEMACH) would be commissioned, and alongside this compulsory 'special measures' would also be introduced. The midwives were told that they must be 'doing something that is causing women to make dangerous decisions about their care', and that this was most likely happening when the women were about 36 weeks pregnant, at an antenatal appointment known as the 'Birth Talk', when women and their midwives met to discuss their options for birth. Becky later commented:

> 'those first allegations against us included the women. If you like, it was about the women almost being given permission by us to behave badly and make bad decisions, dangerous decisions that were then going to kill their babies or damage their babies.'

The Trust had decided to put in place observation and surveillance of all Birth Talks with women with identified risk factors, to be carried out by the two King's consultant midwives. In a strange twist, both the consultant midwives tasked with monitoring the Birth Talks had previously worked in the Albany Practice.

This plan was conveyed to the midwives as a fait accompli, but was this really the case? The midwives had been given absolutely no prior information about any concerns. The planned measures were presented as a way forward that had already been decided. However, astonishingly, having told the midwives about these planned measures, the panel then asked 'Unless you have a better idea?'.

Did those present really have an agreed plan? And how could the midwives possibly have been expected to have a 'better idea' when all of this had just been sprung on them?

The midwives left the meeting room feeling bewildered, upset, and full of questions. The atmosphere in the meeting had felt so hostile, and the midwives had been so shocked, that they had found it impossible to respond. Becky had tried to challenge the figures, but where had they come from? Who had collected them and why? And if they were true, were the Albany midwives really dangerous practitioners? They knew that they had always kept careful records of their outcomes, and that these had been recognised as outstanding both nationally and internationally. The picture was confusing to say the least. What exactly was going on?

Margaret Jowitt
Former editor of Midwifery Matters

The Albany arose out of the Association of Radical Midwives (ARM) vision for the future of maternity care which was published in 1986. ARM envisaged a collective of autonomous midwives working together to care for local women and having a visible presence on the high street. The Albany provided maternity care as midwives and mothers knew it should be provided. Its loss was nothing short of a tragedy for women, babies and families.

The Albany was a warm glow in my heart as I was editing ARM's magazine, *Midwifery Matters*, at the turn of the millennium. It was tangible proof that it was possible to have safe midwife-led, woman-centred maternity care in the 21st century. The Albany was the jewel in the crown of NHS birth services, run by women for women, operating outside of interventionist obstetric practices. It was safe, effective, and loved so much that 2,000 women and families marched to try and save it. Human relationships are paramount in healthcare; a person who knows you, cares for you. Trust is everything.

ARM's vision was used extensively in the Winterton Report of 1992, which itself morphed into *Changing Childbirth* in 1993, becoming government policy. After the Changing Childbirth Implementation Team had ceased to exist, the Albany continued.

As an avid reader of maternity statistics, I would challenge anyone to disagree with my impression that their record for safety and satisfaction dwarfed that of any service anywhere in the country – how could medical management bear to live with a service which had outcomes so much better than their own?

It saddens me how long it took for the news about the allegations against the Albany to filter out: this wonderful group of midwives had lived with allegations about malpractice for getting on for a year before anyone else knew. I was devastated when I found out and rushed up to London for a meeting to find out what on earth had happened and to support in any way I could. I used the pages of *Midwifery Matters* to delve into the intricacies of the allegations from every angle: What is HIE? How should clinical audit be conducted? And that notoriously flawed report, the London Report, undertaken by CMACE, which although it was part of the Confidential Enquiries failed to use the confidential enquiry methodology. A travesty. I am angry to this day. The Albany worked for over 12 years and could work again. We could have an Albany in every town.

How does this relate to maternity services today? Continuity of carer, a woman cared for by a known midwife who is one of a small team, is maternity services policy but is still struggling to survive, the main problem being control of midwives from the central maternity unit. Hospital needs always take precedence over individual women and their babies. For safe maternity care you need to take the midwives out of the hospital (and, if necessary, the hospital out of the midwives) so that the hospital becomes once again a haven for women who need the help of doctors.

The Albany worked. We need it to rise again.

2
From small beginnings...

The seeds of the Albany Midwifery Practice were sown in the early 1990s when a small group of midwives came together in south-east London. Becky was one of those midwives. Having trained as a nurse in the early 1970s, and then having had her own four children in the 1970s and 1980s, she had seen at first hand the state of the maternity services at that time. Home birth had all but disappeared, induction of labour was at an all-time high, and new technologies were creeping into maternity care. She was denied the option of a home birth with her first baby on the spurious grounds that her feet were too small, but went on to have her following three babies at home, the last two with her friend Caroline Flint as her midwife. This experience opened her eyes to the importance of women having a known midwife throughout their pregnancy, birth and in the first weeks with their new baby. Becky trained as an antenatal teacher at the end of the 1970s, but quickly realised that in order to help to change the system she needed to become a midwife herself. During her training, which she did while her children were young, she was in despair about the fragmentation of care experienced by women. After qualifying as a midwife in 1989, she decided to work as an independent midwife until such time as a model of care that she believed in could be set up within the NHS.

Becky was part of a group of independent midwives who started working together in south-east London in the early 1990s. They were all passionate about providing the very best midwifery care they could, and felt strongly that that care should be freely available to all. They began to formulate a midwifery model of care that could work within the NHS. They believed that getting to know a woman during her pregnancy and looking after her during birth and afterwards would lead to improved outcomes for mothers and babies, and would also be more satisfying for midwives. Working independently meant that they were paid by the woman herself for their services, were able to work more autonomously, and were able to provide the one-to-one care they felt was so important for women, babies and families. None of the midwives believed in working privately. Initially they operated a sliding scale, so that payments from wealthier women in their care enabled them to provide care to women with fewer means, until they could find a way to provide their care through the NHS.

The midwives had witnessed through their own practice that continuity of carer increased the normal birth rate and breastfeeding rates, and led to a low intervention rate. Some recent research had also shown that this way of working could improve outcomes for mothers and babies considered to be 'low risk'. They wanted to see if their way of working could improve outcomes for women living in an inner-city area with high levels of deprivation. They also wanted to collect outcome data from all the women they cared for, regardless of obstetric, medical or social 'risk'. In 1993 an opportunity to implement their model of care arose with the publication of *Changing Childbirth*, a government report looking at the evidence collected by an Expert Maternity Group.

Changing Childbirth came to fruition when it did because of women's and midwives' widespread dissatisfaction with maternity services, which came to a head during the 1970s and 1980s. From having been seen as a normal healthy process, which often happened at home, with the woman surrounded by her family and looked after by a community midwife she knew, birth had gradually moved into hospitals until home birth had almost disappeared. In hospitals women were looked after by midwives and doctors they'd never met before. More and more women felt that they were being treated like cattle, as they waited together in antenatal clinics in large groups to be seen by a doctor. In those clinics midwives were overseen by doctors and only allowed to carry out routine care such as checking the women's urine and blood pressure. Women also felt they were on a 'production line' as they entered the hospital in labour, were told to change into a hospital gown, and then required to have a pubic shave and an enema, followed by a bath. Many women had their labours induced or speeded up by having their waters broken or a drug given through a drip inserted into their arm, were confined to bed and attached to fetal heart monitors, and often given pain-relieving drugs whether they asked for them or not. In many places it was routine at that time for women's perineums to be cut (episiotomy) as their babies were being born. After birth new mothers were put in large postnatal wards, their babies were separated from them and kept in nurseries, and brought to their mothers every four hours to feed. Partners were only allowed to visit for a few hours each day.

As early as the 1950s women and midwives had started to get together to question the increasing medicalisation of birth, and several campaigning groups were formed. The National Childbirth Trust (NCT), originally called the Natural Childbirth Trust, was started by Prunella Briance in 1956, and the Association for Improvements in the Maternity Services (AIMS), originally called the Society for the Prevention of Cruelty to Pregnant Women, was formed by Sally Willington in 1960. Both women were concerned about the growing medicalisation of birth, and felt strongly that women should be treated with respect and dignity in childbirth. The Association of Radical Midwives (ARM) was started in 1976 by a group of student midwives, also worried about how women were being treated during pregnancy and how medicalised birth had become. And in 1980 Janet Balaskas' Active Birth Movement came into being, deliberately given that name to challenge the recent medical concept of 'active management of labour'. Active management meant controlling birth as much as possible, with the inevitable interventions necessary to attempt to ensure a labour lasting less than 12 hours.

These campaigns gathered momentum, and in the early 1990s a government health committee was set up to look at maternity services. As well as talking with obstetricians, the committee also asked parents and campaigners for their views and experiences and incorporated these into the report. The 1992 Winterton Report reflected women's views and was hailed by parents, childbirth activists, midwives and some doctors as recognising the need for a less medicalised approach to childbirth. It emphasised that maternity services should be organised around the individual needs of women and families and recognised the impact of poverty on women's and babies' lives. This report had the potential to transform maternity care.

The government then set up an Expert Maternity Group, chaired by Lady Julia Cumberlege (Parliamentary Under Secretary of State for Health), to look at the Winterton Report and draw up a more detailed document for maternity services managers and practitioners, setting out what maternity services should look like. The *Changing Childbirth* report, published in 1993, emphasised the need for choice, control and continuity of care (the 'three Cs') and called for experimental schemes to be set up within the NHS, to put these 'three Cs' into action.

Following the *Changing Childbirth* report, South East Thames Regional Health Authority decided to fund the setting up of three midwifery group practice pilot projects, with the aim of implementing the report's recommendations. The group of independent midwives working together in south-east London was successful in its bid to become one of these projects. They formed the South East London Midwifery Group Practice, known as SELMGP.

So far, so good. However, SELMGP was the only pilot site that was not already funded by an NHS Hospital Trust, and the only money available to it at that time was the £30,000 'set-up' money that had been awarded by the Health Authority. This would clearly not cover the midwives' salaries, and they embarked on a lengthy and complicated negotiation process with the local health authorities in an effort to secure enough NHS funding to support this exciting new model of midwifery care. Progress was painfully slow; initial funding for the care of only 70 women was secured, eventually increasing to provision for 150 women in the first year. In the face of such clear determination, the Health Authority managed to find a pot of money that had been earmarked for 'Health Gain', and an arrangement was made with the practice to use this money for women who might not otherwise have found it easy to access maternity care.

Setting up the practice was exciting, but for the midwives involved it was also financially precarious. With not enough money to support themselves in the beginning, they jointly made the bold decision to work for a year on half pay, in order to get their dream practice up and running. They were acutely aware that this could be a defining moment in the history of midwifery, and felt very strongly that it was 'now or never'. And they were determined not to miss the moment.

The midwifery group was unique and pioneering in so many ways: it formed a partnership, became self-employed, set up a direct contract with the local Health Authority, and undertook to provide a continuity of carer model of midwifery. The midwives found a group of rooms with a shop front in the Albany Community

SELMGP shop front, 1994

Centre in Deptford, south-east London, to act as their base. This ensured easy direct access to the practice, without the need to visit a GP first. They invited senior midwives, obstetricians and eventually also women using the service to form a steering group to monitor the ongoing progress of SELMGP. None of this had been done before, and the midwifery group hoped that it would serve as an NHS model for midwifery care that could be replicated across the country.

SELMGP's innovative way of working gradually developed over the first two years of its existence. The group consisted of six midwives who shared the same commitment to continuity of carer and choice about how and where women had their babies. They worked in pairs in a defined geographical area, so that they could support and cover for each other. Jackie Moulla, who had just completed her midwifery training and had two young children, described joining the practice:

> 'a joy going from the NHS three-year training to a group that was supportive. And the flexibility of working as and when you needed to as opposed to having to go to work at half past seven in the morning whether there were women there or not, and you know, the support from experienced midwives in a group where you're supported and enabled to be a midwife. It was a real community for the midwives and the women.'

Serving some of the most vulnerable women in a deprived inner-city area, the midwifery group quickly became very popular with the local women. Anne, a social worker, staffed the shop front, which looked out onto the busy local market. She offered free pregnancy testing, counselling and termination support, as well as referral to the midwives for midwifery care. Once booked, each woman was then looked after by two named midwives from the practice throughout her pregnancy until her baby was a month old, with both midwives aiming to attend the birth. The midwives provided all the woman's midwifery care, regardless of medical,

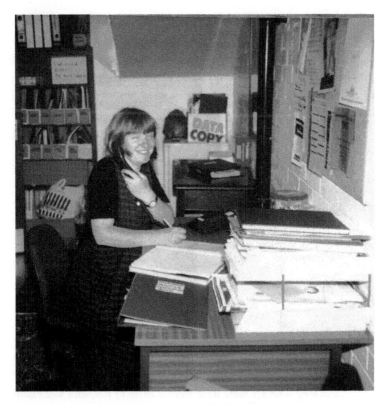

Anne working at the SELMGP

obstetric or social complications. Also embedded in the model were the weekly antenatal and postnatal groups, where women came to discuss, learn and share. The midwives worked with several local hospitals, medical staff and other support services to make sure that the women received all the information, advice, care and support that they needed for their individual circumstances. And crucially, the midwives began to collect data on their outcomes: they wanted to continually monitor and improve their care, as well as eventually show the safety and effectiveness of this way of working.

The group attracted interest around the world for its innovative approach to midwifery care and its excellent outcomes for mothers and babies. It became a resource and an inspiration for midwives and others who wanted to improve care for mothers and babies in their areas and soon became nationally and internationally acclaimed as ground-breaking.

Jane Sandall CBE RM PhD
Professor of Social Science and Women's Health

I first worked with the South East London Midwifery Practice (SELMGP) in 1994. The Practice was one of the case studies for my PhD on how transformational change outlined by *Changing Childbirth* could be achieved and sustained. SELMGP at that time had a pioneering contract with South East Thames Health Authority and later, as the Albany Midwifery Practice, with King's College Hospital. In 2001 and 2008 I worked on evaluations of the Albany Practice, which showed consistently improved outcomes in an area of high social disadvantage with an ethnically diverse population.

What have we learnt from the Albany model? And what is its legacy? We learnt about the importance of self-organisation; of being based in, and engaged with, a local community, of supportive relationships with all healthcare professionals in the community and in the hospital. We learnt about the importance of a 'space of one's own', to run clinics, and hold groups. We learnt about the importance of keeping one's own data on cases and outcomes, of reflection and sharing knowledge, and how to manage out-of-hours work. We learnt about the profoundly positive impact on women and their families of this social model of midwifery, and the importance of midwives using the opportunity that pregnancy brings to make sure that women are embedded in networks of support from families, friends and communities long after the midwifery care ends.

Whose side are you on? We learnt that advocating for women is not a comfortable place to be when colleagues and organisations expect you to be on their side. We learnt about the importance of having champions at a high level and throughout the organisation, and we learnt about how organisations manage reputational risk by focusing on blaming individual health care practitioners and women's behaviour rather than on examining the risk to women's safety from the organisations themselves. We have seen this again and again in investigations of maternity services.

What is the legacy? The model of care that Albany embodied has informed maternity care in many countries: Canada, Australia and the UK in particular. Continuity of care and the importance of relational care from a small group of midwives is advocated currently in Better Births in England and a focus on community-based models is advocated in the 2019 NHS (England) Long Term Plan. Resources have been provided to support implementation and aspirations are high. Much research has shown benefits for women and there is a renewed interest in place-based care and a public health model. The challenging nature of this transformative way of working does not fit organisational ways of doing things. We still have so much to learn about how to successfully implement good humane maternity care, both for women and for those who care for them.

3

Negotiating a contract: not 'can we?' but 'how can we?'

During the winter of 1996–97 the midwives who had formed SELMGP had a visit from their contracts manager at the Health Authority. He was young and nervous and came with bad news. There had been a massive overspend by the Health Authority the previous financial year, and a decision had been taken to cut the funding for many of its smaller projects. SELMGP was one of these. He was very apologetic and said that he recognised what good work the practice was doing, but there was absolutely no room for negotiation.

The midwives were shaken, as they hadn't seen this coming. But they believed absolutely that the model of care that they were pioneering was the way forward for maternity care, and they were not going to let it be destroyed by lack of funding. They vowed to find an answer, and quickly.

The obvious solution was to try and negotiate a contract with the hospital in whose catchment area they were already working. This was Guy's Hospital, and the midwives approached the Head of Midwifery there, hopeful that she would be willing to support the idea. If it were possible, the midwives could remain based at the Albany Centre in Deptford, and continue with the valuable work that they had started in the local community. Women were already coming back to the practice for their second babies, or coming along because they had heard from their friend, or sister, or neighbour, about the care that the midwives were offering. The midwives felt that the set-up had so many benefits: the welcoming walk-in 'office', the direct referral to the midwives, the physical space with rooms available for antenatal checks, meetings and pregnancy and postnatal groups, and the model of midwifery care that was so popular with both the women and the midwives.

However, there was another stumbling block: the Head of Midwifery at Guy's decided not to support a contract with the hospital. So the midwives came together and put their thinking caps on. One of the members of the SELMGP steering group was Cathy Warwick, the recently appointed Head of Midwifery at King's College Hospital in the adjoining borough. Cathy had taken over the post from Janette Brierley, who had already begun to set up what were known as midwifery 'group practices', each with their own particular area of specialisation. The SELMGP midwives decided to approach Cathy Warwick with a proposal to become another King's group practice, but with a radically different model of care.

Cathy Warwick remembers the enthusiastic group of midwives coming to see her, and how this felt:

> 'When that group of people came to me and said "Can you make this happen?" it seemed sensible to try and make it happen. Because here was a group of people who were really committed to something, and who already had a track record...'

She describes how the idea of the model of care felt to her: 'I liked it. It felt right. It felt instinctively important to me. There was something in my psyche which just really felt this was important, and I wanted to continue it'. And Cathy was aware of course that, as well as fitting with her own philosophy of maternity care, it also fitted policy-wise. But could she convince others at King's to make it work, both financially and practically?

It turned out that she could. She describes a feeling of general support for the project, a feeling that 'people didn't want it to go down the tubes', and a possible feeling that the Health Authority might have been 'a bit embarrassed' at their inability to continue funding a service that was successful, popular and valuable. Support was also forthcoming from the Human Resources Director at King's, and from at least one of the senior obstetricians. So for Cathy, it felt like there was an atmosphere of 'Hooray, there's somebody out there who's willing to find a solution to this'. Financially it seems that the Health Authority in fact offered some funding to King's towards the project, and finding the rest of the money 'felt like a no-brainer', as there would always be money available because of vacancies in the maternity department. It was agreed that a certain amount would be taken out of the maternity budget to fund the new group practice, and Cathy was able to argue for the payment to be based around a senior midwife's pay scale, on the basis that (because of its self-managed status) the hospital would not be bearing all the usual employment costs.

Cathy found it wasn't hard for her to contend that 'this was a good thing', and she doesn't remember meeting a huge amount of opposition from anyone, or any real difficulty. However, when it came to putting together a contract, she says 'things got quite tricky'. Nevertheless, Cathy's positive and enabling philosophy of not 'can we?' but 'how can we?' continued to move things forward. Given that this was an entirely new concept, putting together the contract with the hospital was a cutting-edge task. 'We were absolutely making it up as we went along', Cathy says, 'there was nothing to direct us.' However, it turned out that in the end there was only one substantial difficulty, and that was the midwives' absolute insistence on retaining their self-employed and self-managed status, while at the same time being subject to the same policies and protocols ('rules') as all the employed midwives working at King's (this self-employed, self-managed contract model was similar to that of GPs in the UK at the time). Thanks to some committed people working on it, the problem was overcome, and a ground-breaking contract between King's Healthcare NHS Trust and the Albany Midwifery Practice was finally drawn up. The contract was titled 'Agreement for provision of maternity care', and was signed by both parties on 1 April 1997, amid an atmosphere of celebration. On this exciting and historic day for midwifery it truly felt that a new era had begun.

For the midwives it had been imperative to include in the

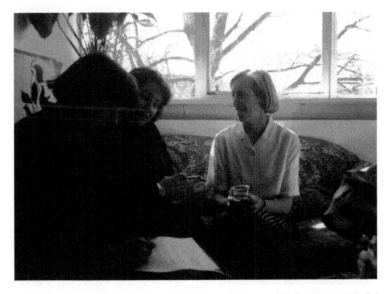

The contract is signed by members of the Albany Practice and Cathy Warwick (right)

contract that they would be caring for a non-selective caseload of local women. To be 'non-selective' the midwives suggested that they could look after women either from a defined geographical area, or women referred to them by one or more designated GP practices, in the area of Peckham in south-east London. They had been collecting their clinical outcomes from the start of the SELMGP project, and were determined to prove that their model of care would lead to improved outcomes for women and babies, and greater satisfaction for women and midwives, even with a non-selective caseload in an area of deprivation. It was agreed that the majority of the women in the midwives' caseload would be referrals from a group of GPs based on the North Peckham estate, which was a perfect solution. In 2019 Peckham, one of the most ethnically diverse areas of the UK, was voted 'the 11th coolest place to live on earth' by *Time Out* London, but in 1997 things were very different. The North Peckham housing estate had become known as one of the most deprived residential areas in western Europe, an archetypal London 'sink estate', with high crime rates and an entrenched gang culture. The killing of Damilola Taylor, a 10-year-old Nigerian boy, in November 2000 became national news. Damilola died on the estate after being attacked by two other young boys. This was the area where the midwives worked, and the stairwell where he was found bleeding to death also led to the home of one of the pregnant women they were caring for at the time.

During the contract negotiations, it was difficult to agree on the perfect number of women to be looked after each year by a 'whole time equivalent', or 'full caseload' midwife. The midwives would be responsible for, and on call all the time for, the women in their caseload, which meant that their working hours would be very different and much more flexible than the usual model of care, where midwives are contracted to work a certain number of set hours each week. This flexibility meant that the midwives would aim to attend the births of all the women they had booked and cared for antenatally. They could also arrange antenatal and postnatal visits with women at mutually convenient times, sometimes in the evening or at weekends. Cathy Warwick was keen that a full caseload Albany midwife should look after 40 women each year, but the midwives felt that they should learn from Lesley Page. As Head of Midwifery at Queen Charlotte's Hospital in London, Lesley had recently initiated and overseen a continuity of carer project known as 'One-to-one', and she was clear that a caseload of 40 women had proved to be too many. So after much use of the 'broken record' technique it was finally agreed that the Albany midwives would have an annual caseload of 36 women each, and this was enshrined in the wording of the contract:

> 'The "Practice" agrees to provide maternity services for 36 women per whole time equivalent midwife per year belonging to the lists of one of the listed GPs.'

With a planned 12 weeks of holiday each year, this meant that each midwife would be on call for approximately four births each month as a primary midwife, and four more as a second midwife.

The contract also allowed the potential for midwives to work in the Practice who would prefer to have fewer women in their caseload, thus enabling them to work fewer hours.

The contract specified broadly what care the midwives would provide for each woman. This included a first booking appointment, care throughout pregnancy, antenatal and postnatal groups, arrangements for tests, scans and any other appointments needed by the woman, care in labour and birth (either at home or in the maternity unit) and postnatal care up to 28 days after birth.

> 'The service will be provided on a 24 hour basis 52 weeks of the year and midwives from the "Practice" will be available to women at all times via pager or telephone.'

The signing of this unprecedented contract really was a ground-breaking event, and it seems extraordinary now that there was very little fanfare at the time. Denis Walsh (then Associate Professor of Midwifery) described the idea as 'amazingly innovative', and Sarah Davies (then Senior Lecturer in Midwifery), described it as 'an idea whose time had come'.

Dame Cathy Warwick

The closure of the Albany Practice was a sad moment for me.

Throughout my career as a midwife I have always believed that the quality of care women receive within maternity services could be enhanced if they were able to access care based on continuity of carer. I have also always believed that all women should receive this, within a service which is free at the point of access. However, I also recognised when I was managing maternity services that, despite my strong support for flexible pay/working patterns, it was a challenge to enable the flexibility that midwives need if they are to deliver such a model within the NHS. It therefore struck me that one way forward was to enable a self-managed model embedded within the regulatory rather than the employment structure of the NHS.

Perhaps there were some who always thought I was on a hiding to nothing, but having set up the Albany model at King's and having watched two other similar models develop in the UK I felt that, although not all midwives would be prepared or able to work in this way, many would, and this could be one way forward. Not the only way but one way. When I was involved with the writing of the *Better Births* report (first published in 2016) and clear evidence had emerged as to the benefits of continuity of carer models, it seemed to me we had a real opportunity to embed such models within the NHS.

I completely understand that every model of care must ensure that all mothers and babies have the best possible outcomes, and every model of care has to be open to scrutiny, challenge and learning, and be prepared to change on the basis of this. As I was not directly involved at the time, I won't ever know for certain why the Albany Practice was closed. All I can imagine is that the reasons were complex, and have to be attributed widely rather than to any one aspect of the model or the system if we are to ever have another 'shot' at this.

Looking back, what I can say for sure is that I am proud that under the care of the Albany Practice so many women received the quality of care to which I will always argue all women should be entitled.

4

Shock, disbelief and confusion

At the end of the meeting at King's in December 2008 which had been so shocking for the midwives, the RCM representative, Carol, had commented that the way the meeting was managed was 'very bad' and that it 'could have been dealt with much better.' Following the meeting Carol had to leave and the midwives, who were all very upset, needed time to think. Carol promised to send the midwives a copy of her minutes as soon as possible. They all agreed to meet in a local cafe early the next day to go over the minutes together and check that everyone had heard and understood what had been said.

The midwives needed to try and make sense of the accusations that were being levelled at them. Following the meeting some of them were crying, and all were in shock. They found it hard to believe that what had been suggested about their practice could be true; they had always kept an ongoing record of their outcomes, and they knew that overall these were excellent. Where had this come from? Who had prompted it and why?

What was also confusing was that the people making the accusations across the table that day included many who had always supported the Albany model of care. The midwives felt a strong sense of betrayal, and were shocked and upset that no one had been in touch or said a word about their concerns before calling them to the meeting. Katie, the Head of Midwifery, was a long-time supporter of the Practice and had also been a Supervisor of Midwives for some of the midwives during the time span of the Case Series. At the time of the meeting, Katie was still Becky's midwifery supervisor. The role of supervisor, which no longer exists in midwifery, involved providing support and advice to midwives to 'ensure their practice is consistent within the regulatory framework'. Katie had even previously sent a Christmas card to the Practice addressing the midwives as 'Albany

Angels', and not long before this had enquired about becoming an Albany midwife herself. Leonie was the Practice's link obstetrician and had been working closely with the midwives for several years, supporting them whenever a woman needed obstetric input into her care. As Natalie said:

> 'the relationship with Leonie really was special wasn't it? It felt like such mutual respect. She knew we would use our heads and do our homework, and be well informed and not call her unnecessarily but it was so reassuring to have someone with her experience to call if needed.'

Leonie had also praised the midwives in a speech at a celebration party for the Albany Practice only the year before. Jill, Consultant Midwife, had helped to found the original South East London Midwifery Group Practice and had remained a personal friend of the Albany. She had also authored a King's Public Health report the previous year, which highlighted the Practice's contribution to improving health outcomes for disadvantaged women and their babies. Jean, Community Manager, had no personal or professional links with the Practice but had always been friendly and supportive. It was only Tony Davies, Consultant Obstetrician and Risk Management Lead, who had ever been less than positive about the Albany model of care.

The morning after the meeting, when the midwives met with Carol over breakfast, she brought along her draft minutes and read them out, promising that later she would write them up and email them to everyone. She confirmed that in the meeting Becky had questioned the accuracy of the Case Series, and had asked for the data to be checked before any further actions were taken. This breakfast meeting with Carol was a friendly get-together over coffee and croissants, and the midwives took comfort from the fact that their union representative was wholeheartedly supporting them. Together they discussed the accusations against the midwives, the document that had been presented, and the actions that the management was proposing. It all seemed rather surreal.

The midwives were feeling numb with shock, but also frantic about what they could possibly do next to try and stop what already seemed to be set in motion. There was no suggestion that they should stop working, so they all needed to continue with their midwifery work, visiting women, attending births, and carrying on the day-to-day life of their very busy Practice.

In the afternoon following the meeting with Carol, two of the midwives, Becky and Danielle, had arranged to meet Kate Brintworth, Danielle's Supervisor of Midwives. They had contacted her for support as soon as they could, and she had suggested that they meet to discuss the situation. Kate, who had very recently been promoted to a senior role at King's as Matron of Community Services, said that she had been told of the concerns about the Practice and had herself questioned the validity of the Case Series. She said she had urged management not to use the Case Series document as she felt it was unprofessional and didn't seem to be accurate:

> 'I remember Linda Sherratt [Midwifery Risk Manager] coming and showing me that they had identified a "cluster" – for want of a better word – and me saying something along the lines of "That's explosive… but are you absolutely sure of the ground you're standing on?… you need to make sure that you've checked and re-checked."'

For the midwives, the days following the meeting were a mix of midwifery work and discussion and planning how to deal with what had just happened. Pauline Armstrong, the Practice Manager (who had not been asked to attend the original meeting) began the enormous task of coordinating communication, as well as doing everything she could to support the midwives. During the next two weeks, in chance meetings with Leonie Penna, a few of the midwives reported that she was very upset and concerned, apologetic but also feeling 'under immense pressure' in her role as their link consultant. She also disclosed that Katie had not been truthful in the initial meeting when she said that nobody else knew about the accusations, as all the consultants knew. She talked about gossip within the unit, and about the fact that some of the other consultants 'wanted more done' (probably stopping all home births). She herself wanted to support the midwives, while at the same time suggesting the possibility of there being a 'groupthink mentality' within the Practice; in other words inferring that a shared (and possibly unchallenged) midwifery philosophy might have led to poor quality decision-making. Looked at in this way, the 'groupthink mentality' could equally have been applied to the group of obstetricians at King's. As Lesley Page aptly commented, 'actually groupthink is a shared philosophy'.

Leonie was clearly feeling compromised, and as the link consultant to the Practice was also implicated in the situation. She told one of the midwives that what was happening 'impacted on her' too. She expressed this dilemma in an email in early January to Katie, Cathy and Jill:

> 'I am in a distinct minority in my belief that the Albany team can be safely allowed to continue to care for pregnant women, with most of my colleagues wanting greater sanctions. To the point that many of them would like home births, if not all births, to be suspended.'

It was clear that this issue was causing profound disagreement and distress to many, not least to Leonie, the consultant obstetrician with whom the midwives had been working so closely for so long.

A letter signed by Katie and Leonie arrived at the Practice six days after that first fateful meeting, confirming that 'certain conditions are to be placed on your practice for the period during which an external review is carried out'. These included the close monitoring of Birth Talks by consultant midwives Jill Demilew and Cathy Walton, discussing birth plans with an obstetrician, and the care of women in labour in hospital being reviewed by an obstetrician 'at regular intervals'. The letter also informed the Practice that an outside body had already been approached 'to undertake a review of all the cases where there was a poor outcome', and that this review might take up to a year to complete. The letter ended with an apology for this being a 'source of anxiety for you all', and stated 'we have no choice but to address these concerns in this way'. Lesley Page, Professor of Midwifery, later described these measures put in place by King's as something similar to 'a totalitarian regime, you know, when you go in and kind of watch people and spy on them'.

The midwives and Pauline were spending all their waking hours agonising about how best to deal with what had been thrown at them. They were convinced that there had to be more to the story. Above all they were deeply concerned about the Case Series, which, quite literally, didn't add up. About a week after the initial meeting Becky was staring at the numbers for the umpteenth time when she noticed a disparity in the totals on the front page. Numbers that actually added up to 10 were documented as 12, and percentages were wrongly calculated in favour of the hospital (and at the expense of the Albany). In a private conversation with a senior public health consultant a few weeks later, Becky was told 'Your reputation is being besmirched based on a dodgy little report'. Professor Nicky Leap, from the University of Technology, Sydney, recalls that when she first saw the Case Series, she immediately noticed that most of the babies included were born in hospital under medical care, and she thought that the list of cases was an example of 'appropriate transfer' by the midwives. It was clear to nearly everyone who laid eyes on it that the Case Series document was an unprofessional and unreliable piece of work.

Pauline's mind was also whirring. She very quickly put together the following list of comments and questions, which would subsequently be sent to Katie as agenda items for a meeting in the New Year:

> '1. We have several questions on the way the data presented has been collected and analysed. We believe there to be serious flaws in the collection, not least over which babies are included in the data.
> 2. We wonder why you have chosen this period – 2 years and 7 months – is there significance to these dates?
> 3. We would like to know what correlations are being drawn from

the data, how this analysis has taken place and what you believe to be significant.

4. Each of the cases you have highlighted on your list has already been scrutinised by King's risk management process. We would like to see the reports of each of these cases.

5. Given that a majority of these babies were born in hospital we wonder if you have looked at the role of all team members in the babies' care.

6. What is your definition of significant risk?

7. Why was the meeting called with such short notice and in such a secretive way, using our personal mobiles and even calling in one midwife from holiday?

8. Why were no minutes taken of this meeting by King's?'

Carol, the RCM representative, had gone quiet. There was no communication from her, and no sign of the minutes that she had promised to send as soon as possible. Because of this, it was decided that a higher level of union representation was needed.

Pauline contacted the Royal College of Midwives' Regional Officer, Francine Allen, saying: 'Midwives in the Practice are really struggling at the moment, very upset and very low morale as you can imagine'. With Francine's help Pauline wrote a reply to the letter from Katie and Leonie, attaching her list of comments and questions, and proposing a meeting at the Practice on 15 January 2009 with Francine present. In the letter she commented:

> 'We would like to express our shock and dismay about the allegations against us. The wellbeing of mothers and babies is our primary consideration and we are hugely concerned at the notion of harm coming to babies as a result of our care. In particular we are requesting to discuss the data, the process of your enquiry, the statistics and the concerns and contents of your letter.'

Everyone's minds kept coming back to the Case Series. What was going on? How could such a reputable organisation be threatening one of their own trusted midwifery group practices based on such poor quality calculations? Pauline contacted Jane Sandall, Professor of Midwifery and Women's Health at King's College London, asking her for comments on the Case Series document. Jane and colleagues immediately saw the inadequacies in the data collection and presentation, and drew up and sent to the Practice suggestions for a different way of collecting and analysing the data.

Within two weeks of the meeting on 3 December, Jill and Cathy, the Consultant Midwives, visited the Practice to discuss the monitoring of the Birth Talks. It was suggested that one or other of them would attend four Birth Talks with each midwife, during which they would document their observations using an agreed process. Once finished, they would write a report to feed back to the Head of Midwifery.

At the same time as the monitoring of the Birth Talks was getting underway, Sarah Dawson, new in post as the Divisional General Manager for Women and Children, felt it important to update other senior obstetric and neonatal consultants and supervisors of midwives on the 'Albany review'. She emailed them a week before Christmas calling an urgent meeting. The email, which was subsequently leaked to the midwives, was titled 'Emergency Meeting', and showed just how deeply felt were the concerns in the maternity department. It was clear that not only was there real anxiety about the safety of the Albany Practice, but also concerns about how the issue was being addressed. There was obviously a feeling that all Albany women were now potentially in danger, not just those with 'identifiable risk factors'.

Following this meeting Katie wrote the following email to everyone who had attended:

> 'Dear All
> Thank you so much for coming to this meeting on Friday morning. It was helpful to share how we had proposed to manage this issue and to hear your concerns relating to factors you felt were not being addressed particularly well in the proposed review. As a result of

the discussion on Friday, we are going to institute two additional monitoring systems as well as those already being put in place.

To ensure that the "36 week birth talk" is completed to expected standards for all women including low-risk women (for whose talks Cathy and Jill will not be present) Leonie will design a "Contract" document which will detail all the issues to be discussed e.g. place of birth, management of the 3rd stage, resuscitation of the baby at home and in hospital etc. This will be used as a script for the talk and will give risks for each course of action taken. On completion it will be signed by the midwife and the woman. We anticipate this could be used by all the community midwives in the future.

To ensure that when intermittent auscultation is used for low-risk women in the Albany practice, the standard is as in our guidelines, we are designing an assessment tool to use in assessing each of the Albany midwives' practice. The assessment will be carried out by senior midwives (not the coordinators) on the labour ward as soon as is practicable.

We will hear from Cemach in the New Year about the details of the review they are to carry out. Until then we will proceed with the measures detailed here.

This is going to be a very difficult period for us all. I would hope that if you have any other concerns that you will discuss them with Mike Savvas [Clinical Director] *or myself.*

Best wishes

Katie'

Katie subsequently wrote to the Albany midwives on New Year's Eve, advising them of the two further measures 'that I feel I must put in place'. The tone of the letter was friendly, almost apologetic:

'*A number of people present at the [emergency] meeting raised concerns about how we propose to manage any potential risk to Albany women while the external review takes place… The concerns… related to low-risk women and were articulated because a number of Albany women in the last two years have been low-risk but have still had a poor outcome. Those present were made aware of the plans for the consultant midwives to sit in on 36 week birth talks with women who are high risk. But they wanted assurances that low-risk women were also being made aware of the potential risks (however low they may be) of choosing, for example, to birth at home. To try to reassure these individuals, Leonie Penna is working on a document to be used as a framework for the 36 week birth talk which if used will ensure that couples are made aware of the possible consequences of choosing a home birth.*

I am aware that this approach is somewhat unbalanced because we do not inform couples of the risk they take when they choose to birth in hospital. However, I would ask for your tolerance at the present time.'

As well as the monitoring of the Birth Talks, the second measure to be put in place was the assessment of 'how each midwife in the practice monitors a baby using intermittent auscultation.'

Intermittent auscultation is one of the most basic day-to-day skills all midwives are taught in their training. It involves listening to a baby's heartbeat, either with a pinard (a type of wooden ear trumpet) or a hand-held doppler machine, and is common practice in all straightforward labours. For the midwives in the Practice this was part of the bread and butter of midwifery, something they would all have done thousands of times. Katie knew this, and was apologetic: 'I am sorry that this calls into question your capabilities with respect to these fundamental midwifery skills. But to satisfy those who are in doubt, I have agreed that we will assess how each midwife in the practice monitors a baby... This will be done once for each midwife...'. The midwives saw this as demeaning, describing it as 'utter humiliation'. It goes without saying that when these assessments took place no problems were found.

One can only imagine the kind of pressure Katie must have been under in order to agree to the midwives being investigated for the most basic of midwifery skills. It is surely not possible that she could have entertained the idea that skilled midwives working in the community were unable to properly monitor a baby's heartbeat during labour and birth. Did she feel unwilling, unable or frightened to assert a midwifery view on these matters and advocate for midwifery and the midwives? What was happening behind the scenes?

Leonie Penna, meanwhile, was clearly feeling more and more challenged. In her email to Katie, Cathy and Jill, she tried to analyse 'the problem', at the same time as admitting 'I agree that the data set was hastily put together and is not as polished as it could be.' However, she then went on to say 'the numbers are not borderline in their significance and the probability that there is a genuine problem is extremely high.' Discussing the measures put in place, she commented: 'I fully accept that I have no evidence that any of the measures we are introducing are going to make any difference', but then went on to say 'I believe these measures will make a difference… all the proposed measures are something that sends a signal to other concerned colleagues that we are trying to address aspects of the Albany midwives practice that they are concerned about.' Leonie's email concluded: 'I have to add that I am reaching my limits in my ability to support this process and I feel in the middle with dissent on both sides'. This was after all a group of midwives whom she liked, got on well with, trusted and supported (and had even invited to dinner at her house), and who were now under scrutiny based on data that by any standards could not be described as robust.

Not surprisingly, throughout this time the midwives could talk or think about little else other than the situation they found themselves in. Life in the Practice had to carry on, however, with busy days filled with antenatal and postnatal visits, as well as births. Natalie, who had been heavily pregnant at the time of the December meeting, said later to Becky: 'and then in the middle of all of this, you, Fran and Mary were all at Emily's birth for the whole day of the 4th January'. Natalie's birth was long and complicated, and three of the midwives shared the care of their friend and colleague, and the eventual joy at the birth of her baby Emily.

On 10 January Becky was at the third birth of a woman she knew well and whose first two births she had also attended. The labour was taking a while to get going, but as it was a third baby Becky decided to stay and make herself comfortable by the fire in the living room, while Anna moaned along with her contractions in the kitchen. Even though she was in the happy situation of being a midwife to a friend in labour, Becky couldn't get the Albany crisis out of her head. Since Anna didn't need her for the time being, she decided to make a phone call to Cathy Warwick, previous Director of Midwifery at King's and now Chief Executive of the Royal College of Midwives, to see if she had any advice.

On the phone Cathy was very supportive and friendly. Needless to say she knew the Practice well, having set up their initial contract and managed it until only a few months before the December meeting. She said that she thought there were two significant issues: 'is there a problem? And has it been handled correctly?' Cathy told Becky that Katie had been in touch with her prior to the first meeting with the Albany midwives to discuss her concerns, and admitted that she hadn't talked to the midwives. Cathy had expressed her shock at this and suggested strongly to Katie that she talk to the midwives urgently before calling them to a meeting, which Katie never did. Becky and Cathy talked about the way forward, and Cathy suggested that the Practice talk to the Deputy Chief Executive at King's, Jacqueline Docherty, to discuss their concerns about the process. She did however describe Jacqueline Docherty as 'firm and unemotional', and said it would be a good idea to brief her before any meeting.

A meeting with the Deputy Chief Executive seemed like a good idea (if daunting), so this was arranged as a matter of urgency within a few days. Becky had a friend who was working for the Audit Commission* at the time, and she offered to help

---

* The Audit Commission was a statutory public corporation that existed in the UK between 1 April 1983 and 31 March 2015. Its main objective was to appoint auditors to a range of local public bodies in England (including the NHS from 1990), set the standards for auditors and oversee their work. When it closed, its functions were transferred to the private, voluntary or not-for-profit sectors.

write a briefing paper. Following an introduction and some background to the issues, the paper stated:

> 'In our view, the data was incomplete, inaccurate, miscalculated and subjective. We have since asked for clarification around the data but to date this has not been supplied… We understand that the original report (Case Series) was revised one week later to include more cases and also understand that there has been a further revision since this. We have not been officially told of, or seen, either of these revisions and again this raises our concerns about the reliability of the data.'

The midwives and Pauline were hopeful that Jacqueline Docherty would listen sympathetically, and offer some support and guidance for the way forward. The briefing paper concluded:

> 'we have requested this meeting to raise our concerns and ensure you are aware of the issues and the manner in which they have been (and continue to be) handled. We would also seek your support in ensuring openness and transparency in the communication surrounding the issues and the process from now on.'

It was with some trepidation that Pauline, and midwives Zoe and Becky, waited outside Jacqueline Docherty's office on the morning of 14 January 2009. They were nervous about how they would be received, but felt sure that they were doing the right thing. Their intention was to have a confidential discussion with a very senior member of the Trust. This would hopefully be an opportunity to explain the story from their point of view, and to explore the best way to proceed.

They were greeted by Jacqueline Docherty in a friendly enough fashion. She ushered them into her office, and asked them to sit along one side of a large desk. She then disappeared through a door in a corner of the room, and the midwives and

Pauline assumed that she was organising some refreshments. But then both Katie Yiannouzis and Sarah Dawson appeared through the same door. It was immediately obvious that the meeting that the Practice had thought would be confidential was going to be nothing of the sort.

The minutes of the meeting, taken by Pauline, state: 'JD opened the meeting by saying she had invited KY and SD in the interests of transparency. She didn't say, and we neglected to ask, why we hadn't been asked or informed.' The truth was that both the midwives and Pauline were totally taken aback by the appearance of the very people who were implementing a process that they had wanted to discuss privately.

The minutes of the meeting go on to document a discussion about 'the scale of the problem', about the confidential review (CEMACH) into the Albany Midwifery Practice and how it would be organised, and about the 'temporary measures'. Jacqueline Docherty commented 'Perhaps these measures can be reviewed in the future to judge whether they are the right mechanisms'; small comfort for the two midwives present. However, the power dynamic in the room was evident, and it was clear that on the management side of the table conclusions had already been reached.

Katie then talked about the Case Series document. She repeated that over a period of two years and seven months it appeared that a disproportionate number of Albany babies had been admitted to Special Care with HIE. The midwives and Pauline began to protest about the inaccuracies in the data, and then Katie, with little or no apology, produced the *third* version of the Case Series. The midwives had only recently seen a second version, which had been unofficially shown to them eight days earlier. In this third version the numbers of babies documented as having been admitted to the Neonatal Unit with HIE had been changed yet again. The situation was now beyond surreal: it was nightmarish, bizarre and illogical... it felt kafkaesque.

Lesley Page CBE

Visiting Professor in Midwifery Florence Nightingale Faculty of Nursing Midwifery and Palliative care, Adjunct Professor University of Technology Sydney

Albany was iconic. It represented not only life-enhancing high-quality care in the true sense of quality, but was also forward-facing in so many ways. Contracted into the health service around the time of *Changing Childbirth*, Albany fitted all the aspirations for maternity care outlined then, and the model is still central to new government policy for the UK. Looking back over the justifications for closing Albany I was struck by the criticism on the King's website of the positive view of birth promoted by the Albany midwives. Yet that positive view has never been more needed.

Albany is iconic. Its closure to me represented a kind of vandalism. Albany was a well-known example of many closures of services with positive outcomes over the years. The closure, these closures, were something to be grieved over. Moving forward there are so many lessons to be learned. These lessons are highly relevant now. Albany was closed on a skewed idea of safety and how safety is evaluated. How does a skewed idea of safety still prevail, especially now when it runs alongside so many of the most progressive policies around childbirth we have ever known?

Women and babies deserve high-quality safe care around pregnancy and birth, and in the early weeks of life. Yet so much is done in the name of safety that actually causes harm. Birth is a critical and sensitive time, when safety and quality mean not only survival, but also the possibility of strong relationships, hope, love and joy. So much of what masquerades as safety disturbs and prevents the best start. So much of the current approach to safety fills us all with fear.

I am still so sad about the closure of Albany. All we can do now is learn from the model of practice and understand why and how Albany was closed. This will help take us to a better and more hopeful future. Let's fill our future with this hope.

5
The golden years

When Mavis Kirkham, Professor of Midwifery, first learned that the Practice was under threat, she remarked that 'ironically, it is probably the most evaluated midwifery service there is.' Over the years the evaluations had been consistently positive, showing that the Practice not only achieved exceptionally good health outcomes for women and babies, but that the families and midwives also loved it: 'you never feel rushed' and 'when you need help it's always there for you'. There was 'nothing but praise for the excellent care Albany midwives provided', it was 'just brilliant, they were all really good at making you feel at ease'. Looking back, Fran, one of the midwives, commented:

> *'I loved working as an Albany midwife for two reasons. Firstly it meant I could work with women in true partnership and offer them proper choice and support in the journey before, during and after birthing their baby. Secondly it was an absolute joy to go to work every day with the most amazingly supportive midwife colleagues that shared the same philosophy about birth as me.'*

Up until 2008 the Practice was seen as an asset by its own Trust. In the evaluation carried out by King's in 2001,[*] it is stated that 'The presence of Albany reflects well on the Trust externally, and is seen as a factor in recruitment, and staff development'. Local health visitors and GPs were quoted as being very positive about the Practice, and said that they found the women were noticeably more relaxed and confident as new mothers. One health visitor said that you could tell who had had an Albany midwife as soon as you

---

[*] J. Sandall, J. Davies, C. Warwick (2001) *Evaluation of the Albany Midwifery Practice: Final Report* Nightingale School of Midwifery, Kings College London, London.

entered her home because she was more 'relaxed, competent and happier'. And Cathy Warwick, the Director of Midwifery at the time, gave many talks at conferences and seminars in the UK and internationally about this innovative community-based project.

The Albany Practice was viewed as a beacon of good practice by midwifery services around the world, and received acclaim and positive feedback locally, nationally and internationally. Articles extolling the virtue of continuity of carer and how the Albany Midwifery Practice provided this were published in midwifery journals, childbirth journals and in the press. Academics, practitioners and opinion leaders frequently cited it as a model of good practice. There was a constant flow of visiting student midwives from all over the UK and overseas, who found that they finally experienced what they often called 'real midwifery'. Typically they left feeling inspired, and 'with a positive view of midwifery and the benefits that can be gained when women are made the focal point of care.'

Associate Professor of Midwifery Denis Walsh explained that the 'cutting edge' Practice brought together the best of midwifery and 'ticked all the boxes'. Those boxes included improving health outcomes, providing continuity of care from a known and trusted midwife, increasing women's choices, increasing normal birth rates, decreasing interventions and increasing breastfeeding rates, all of which the Albany Practice clearly did. One of the mothers, Rix Pyke, commented on this in a letter to the Practice:

> 'So please remember this: you are a fantastic project, working in a wonderful way and we are SO lucky to have you here in Peckham. You are there at the beginning offering calm, sensible, trusting, positive energy – welcoming babies in with such a light touch. You are leading the way back from bright lights and a slap at birth – to gentle, powerful, loving entry into life. THANK YOU.'

There is now more and more research about the benefits of relationships in healthcare. Recent work has shown that seeing the same GP can dramatically reduce the chance of dying prematurely. This evidence about relational care was not widely known in the late 1990s and early 2000s. The Albany evaluations were some of the first of their kind to show what can be achieved when skilled midwives provide continuity of carer.

The first evaluation in 2001, four years after the Albany Practice opened, showed that compared with women who were looked after by midwives in the other King's College Hospital midwifery group practices, those looked after by the Albany midwives had more normal births, used a birthing pool more often, had fewer elective caesarean sections, used hardly any pain-relieving drugs, and were more likely to breastfeed at birth and for at least the first four weeks of their babies' lives. The conclusion was that the Albany midwives were 'providing a form of maternity care that women feel positive about', that it was 'woman centred' and that they were achieving what they set out to do. That is, to provide a high level of continuity of carer, give women the information they needed to be fully involved in decisions about their care, support normal birth, improve women's experiences of pregnancy and birth, help women to become confident mothers, make maternity care accessible to women who might not otherwise seek out maternity care during their pregnancies, and positively influence the philosophy of care in the Trust as a whole.

Jill Demilew, Consultant Midwife at King's, published a report in 2007 titled *Supporting Wellbeing: Tackling Health Inequality*. It looked at how King's midwifery group practices were contributing to women's wellbeing, reducing the impact of inequalities and increasing choice and continuity of carer. At the time, the priority at King's was to 'provide a choice of safe, high quality maternity care for all women and their partners' and to plan services that would 'address improving outcomes for more vulnerable and disadvantaged families'. This was exactly what the Albany Midwifery Practice had been set up to do. The report found that even though the Practice was looking after women in one of the most deprived areas of England, and included women who had medical, obstetric and social complications, their outcomes were always as good as those of women and babies looked after at King's and in some cases better. For example, the Albany women had fewer very low birthweight or premature babies, and very few Albany babies needed to be transferred to the Neonatal Unit. The women had some of the lowest intervention rates in labour, and their breastfeeding initiation rate was the highest within the Trust.

By 2008 the Practice had looked after over 2,000 women. Professor Jane Sandall and Becky collaborated in a retrospective review, known as 'The 2,000 Women Study', looking at the Practice's birth outcomes over a 10-year period (1997–2007). Data were collected from the birth summary sheets and analysed using a statistical package. Outcomes reported included type and place of birth, rates of analgesia use, perineal trauma, postpartum haemorrhage and breastfeeding. The findings of the study were presented in a paper delivered at the International Confederation of Midwives Congress in Glasgow in June 2008.

The 2,000 Women Study showed the same excellent outcomes as the 2001 evaluation. Normal birth rates remained very high and the caesarean section and instrumental delivery rates remained very low. Despite the Albany being situated in an area with low breastfeeding rates, the rates for Albany women and babies were exceptionally high, with 92 per cent of the women breastfeeding their babies at birth, and 74 per cent still exclusively breastfeeding after four weeks, with an extra 17 per cent of the women mixed feeding. This compares with a national breastfeeding rate at the time of 35 per cent exclusively breastfeeding at one week, and 21 per cent at six weeks. The study also showed that the number of babies dying around the time of birth (known as the perinatal mortality rate) was 4.9 in 1,000. In 2006 in England and Wales it was nearly 8 in 1,000, and in Southwark, where the Albany Practice was situated, it was 11.4 in 1,000 babies in 2003–05.

These are remarkable statistics for some of the most deprived women and babies in the country. The study concluded: 'The data collected has provided a unique opportunity to examine some rarer outcomes, and has demonstrated the quality and safety of caseload midwifery in this setting.'

It seems inconceivable that the midwives were accused of dangerous practice not long after this study was completed. According to the evaluations, there was no reason to think that the Albany Practice was anything but safe and successful. It even managed to improve outcomes for mothers and babies in challenging circumstances – something that has long puzzled researchers, policy-makers and practitioners. It was also innovative and challenged the medical model of birth.

Not everyone at King's, however, was happy about this. Although the Practice was repeatedly shown to be successful, it later transpired that dark clouds had been quietly gathering in the background for some time.

Nicky Leap
Adjunct Professor of Midwifery, University of Technology Sydney

The Albany Midwifery Practice demonstrated to the world what can be achieved when midwives provide continuity of carer to women whose lives are challenged by social disadvantage. The wealth of research evidence about the Practice has identified outstanding outcomes for women and babies and the profoundly positive effect midwifery care from Albany midwives had on women's experiences and lives.

If we pin these remarkable achievements on midwifery continuity of carer alone, we may be missing other important aspects of what we can learn from the Albany Midwifery Practice. The Practice was an important example of a community-based, social model of maternity care, one that addressed the principles underpinning primary health care and public health strategies, particularly around understanding the social determinants of health, building social support and enhancing community participation and empowerment. This way of working is not just about being visible and accessible in the community, although that is an important starting point. It is about a philosophy of midwifery care that seizes every opportunity to reduce social isolation through putting pregnant women and new mothers in touch with each other and with community-based agencies, in order to promote friendships and support.

The story of how NHS funding was secured to promote health gain for women who were seen as being socially disadvantaged is described in this book. This inherently political way of working was first described by the midwives in the South East London Midwifery Group Practice, who were based in a 'walk-in' shop front in the Albany Community Centre in Deptford in the 1990s. I was lucky enough to have been one of those midwives. We embraced any opportunity to engage with people at community events, using posters and pregnancy models as a vehicle for the sharing of information and resources. It was in Deptford that we developed the concept of the 36-week 'Birth Talk' visit in the woman's home, and introduced the idea of bringing women together in antenatal and postnatal groups to support each other and learn from each other's stories. Years later, as a researcher, when interviewing women who had received care from the Albany midwives, I heard the same thing over and again: 'I made friends for life.'

Midwives who work in a similar way to the Albany midwives develop a strong sense of autonomy and group solidarity. They understand the importance of meeting at least once a week as a group to support each other, reflect on events, discuss liaison with other practitioners, and importantly, to explore the uncertainties that often underpin challenges and decision-making about practice. This way of working is such a long way away from the 'risk management' culture of contemporary maternity services. Hopefully this book can offer some understanding of this clash of paradigms, thus informing the development of sustainable, community-based midwifery group practices, underpinned with the same inspirational philosophy as that of the Albany midwives. We can lament the closure of the Albany Midwifery Practice while appreciating and celebrating its precious legacy.

6
Rumblings

The midwives felt that their gold-standard model of care had been hit by a bolt from the blue on that fateful morning of 3 December 2008. The model had political support and excellent outcomes, and the feedback from those served by the Practice was overwhelmingly positive. Yet suddenly it was the subject of an investigation for being potentially dangerous. What could possibly have gone so wrong so quickly? Was there anything that had happened previously that could shed light on the extraordinary turn of events? Digging deeper, and looking back over the history of the Albany at King's, there was clearly more to the story.

The 'bolt' delivered to the Albany Practice arose from both general and specific tensions between a midwifery or social view of birth and a more technological or obstetric view of birth. Given the increasing dominance of obstetrics in maternity care, new midwifery initiatives inevitably gave rise to concerns and dissent. Some researchers, practitioners, politicians and lay people had been expressing concerns about increasing interventions during childbirth, the impact of this on women's agency and wellbeing, and the rising costs involved. This had been discussed at a political level in the early 1990s, and the policy document *Changing Childbirth* (1993) strongly recommended a social, midwifery approach to birth with women as decision-makers.

This subject was raised in the House of Lords in January 2003, in a wide-ranging debate on the quality of provision for maternity services in the UK. Baroness Thomas of Walliswood described being struck by the 'chaos that seems to hang over the service and policy discussions about it' and the 'lack of consensus among practitioners on what constitutes good practice'. She also suggested that: 'There can be no doubt about what women want, once someone gives them a chance to talk', and that this included good advice, continuity of midwifery care and community-based settings for birth. Baroness Noakes also spoke about this:

> 'We have heard from many people this evening that pregnancy and childbirth are not illnesses: they are part of normal human life. Yet maternity services have developed around a different concept. I mean no disrespect to the medical profession, and in particular to obstetricians, when I say that the medicalisation of pregnancy and childbirth is part of today's problems'.

She went on to mention caesarean section rates being 'frighteningly high and still rising', rising rates of instrumental births, anaesthesia use and episiotomy rates: 'It is clear that the rate of normal births is declining. That is not what women want or deserve'. During the debate the Albany Midwifery Practice was cited by Baroness Cumberlege as a model of maternity care to aspire to, and the Earl of Listowel, who had taken the trouble to visit the Practice in preparation for the debate, cited the evaluation report from 2001, and the achievements of the AMP in an area of high deprivation. He extolled the virtues of the Albany model for mothers and babies, and also for the midwives. In a letter to the Practice following his visit he said: 'It has been a great pleasure learning about the important service you provide for mothers in Peckham.' He suggested that such a model would improve parent-child attachment, and 'go some way to ensuring that fewer children go to prison, that fewer children are taken into care and that the cycle of failure from generation to generation is somewhat ameliorated', and at the same time would help with staff recruitment and retention by being 'an incitement for midwives to continue to work in the profession, and to return to the profession, and for young people to train as midwives'.

Even without the weight of research that the years ahead would bring, there was still clear evidence to show that skilled midwifery care and support during childbearing could improve outcomes for women and their babies. Nonetheless, distrust and fear of midwifery skills and initiatives were well documented. This fear is long standing and continues to endure, despite overwhelming evidence now showing that skilled midwifery provides a wide range of health and social benefits to mothers, babies and families.

At the time the Albany story was unfolding there were still many who were sceptical about the idea of midwifery group practices. It is therefore not surprising that not everyone at King's subscribed to the view that the AMP was a gold-standard model, or that some doctors felt uncomfortable about the midwifery group practices at King's. Nor is it surprising that they were feeling increasingly more concerned about the Albany Practice, which stood out at King's due to its high home birth rate. However, the AMP midwives were also working alongside King's doctors and midwives: they attended antenatal appointments with women, supported them during their births in hospital, and visited them postnatally. For some hospital practitioners, this brought to light further concerns. Because the Albany midwives knew the women in their care so well and had had lengthy conversations with them throughout their pregnancies, the women were often clear and assertive about what they wanted. The trusting relationships they had developed enabled the midwives to advocate for them if they were not being listened to or felt unable to make their wishes known. This made both the women and their midwives more visible, and for some King's practitioners, more challenging than other women and midwives. Zoe remembers going into the Special Care Baby Unit (SCBU) and finding a palpable sense of 'bad feeling' from some of the staff there, as though 'we were from *that* Practice' and had somehow caused the baby to be admitted. As Natalie later remembered: 'All midwives were suspect, but especially the group practices, and the Albany were the "Albany Assassins". Do you remember that term? Sends a sick chill through me.'

Some members of the medical staff were so challenged by the Albany midwives' close relationships with women that they wanted the midwives to stop accompanying the women to antenatal obstetric appointments. Mary recalls:

'they wanted us not to go with the women. Because we always went with the women to their obstetric appointments. They wanted us not to go... they wanted the women to go on their own... It didn't happen, but there was discussion that we shouldn't be going. You know, why were we going with the women? We were influencing what was happening in those appointments...'

A journalist whose wife gave birth to their second child with the Albany midwives in 1998 was moved to write about the experience, having picked up some antagonism towards the Albany midwives from the doctor on duty. He explicitly addressed one of the assumptions which was later made by King's and then by the Centre for Maternal and Child Enquiries (CMACE) during the AMP investigations – that the midwives were somehow imposing their own views on women and causing them to make unsafe decisions about their pregnancies and births:

'It is important for you to understand that when [the midwife] said my wife was adamant about a natural birth without forceps, she said so because she knew my wife very well. She did not say so because that was her own preference. She had discussed the options at length with my wife – and I mean at length.'

In 2001, the researchers who carried out the first evaluation of the Practice noted similar background tensions among some of the medical staff. Senior obstetricians seemed supportive, and relationships were generally positive between them and the Practice, but some of the neonatologists were concerned about the outcomes for some of the Albany babies, although they had no data to support their position. Jane Sandall, one of the researchers, recalled:

'So there were beginning to be rumblings. They were worried about outcomes. But when we asked them for the outcome data, they didn't have it because neonatal outcomes are kept on a separate *system to the maternity system. I remember asking them, if you have concerns, why aren't you consistent, why aren't you setting up a data collection system across the whole trust so that you can look at it properly?'*

The researchers also noticed concerns among some of the hospital midwives about the level of midwifery autonomy embedded within the Albany model of care, suggesting that this way of working was detrimental to the midwives' health and wellbeing. Jane Sandall observed:

'you know, you're damned if you do, and you're damned if you don't. So if you go in with a woman and you look tired, then the other midwives will say, "Oh that's a terrible way to work." You know, "They'll burn themselves out." And then if you let it be known that you've been working at home or you've gone shopping this morning, but you're doing an antenatal visit in the evening, they'll say, "Well that's a bit of a doss – they're not working hard enough, are they?" You know, so there was that – whatever you said or did that model would be criticised.'

Pauline Armstrong, the AMP manager, in a similar comment, highlighted the resentment that is not uncommonly shown towards those working in different ways, pointing out that other staff at King's sometimes felt the Albany midwives were doing less because their working patterns were so different. She recalls:

'the Albany always sat slightly uncomfortably at King's. There was huge support there, but there were also quite a lot of midwives who either didn't support the model or were resentful of the model and resentful of the way the midwives came and went on the wards. Perhaps not understanding it and not feeling that the midwives were pulling their weight in some way. So I do think that the Practice itself was not universally welcomed because it was a bit different.'

Cathy Warwick also commented on this, saying that 'what the obstetricians were really scared of was difference'. The Albany midwives were acutely aware of this at times. As Mary said:

> 'I think there was a real kind of mistrust, a definite feeling that we were some kind of other; that we were witchy, or that we were doing things that they couldn't understand. There was something that they couldn't understand about the Practice, therefore they found it disturbing and thought that we must be doing something wrong. And, I think because actually a lot of the women spoke quite powerfully about what they wanted, that it almost felt quite threatening. And I think that people like Mike Marsh [King's obstetrician] really didn't like that, and found that really challenging, and thought that we must be doing something. And hopefully we were doing something. I really hope that we were doing something to make women feel able to say what they wanted'.

The midwives speculated that there was a feeling among the medical staff that they lacked control over the midwives and the women. Professional jealousy may also have come into it, as the AMP increasingly gathered national and international acclaim.

During the years that the AMP held its contract with King's, tensions came and went depending on political influences, changes in maternity services, local circumstance, and roles and personnel at King's. In 2003 a flashpoint occurred, which was almost a precursor to events in 2008. The concerns about outcomes for Albany babies (and those from the other midwifery group practices at King's) that arose every so often gathered momentum and unsurprisingly focused on home births.

Mike Marsh had become the official link obstetrician for the AMP in 2002. Not long after this Cathy Warwick and the midwives noticed that some of the King's obstetricians were showing increasing concern about the community midwifery practices, including the AMP. Cathy described how Mike Marsh, together with another obstetrician, Tony Davies, started keeping a 'list' of every woman and baby booked with the community midwifery practices where the birth was not entirely straightforward. She recalls:

> 'I was very anxious that when serious incidents happened from the practices – and of course they were happening in equal numbers in the hospital – that it would be somehow harder to stop everybody going "It's the practices that are the problem. It's home birth that is the problem." So what I remember is [...] not that there was something wrong with the practices, but that people were increasingly looking for something to be wrong'.

Cathy 'felt anxious walking past his [Tony Davies's] office' on a Monday morning as 'he'd be sitting with another large pile of case notes'. She describes how Mike Marsh and Tony Davies would 'worry away in that office together'.

Mary recalled that when she joined the Practice in 2003, 'there were things going on' with Mike Marsh and one of his colleagues and that he 'kept exploding' that this was another baby coming into King's from the community midwifery practices. Despite Cathy Warwick meeting with him to discuss the situation, his concerns continued to grow, and increasingly focused on Albany mothers and babies. Each time investigations were carried out, however, the care given by the Albany midwives and midwives from other group practices was found to be appropriate. And as Cathy pointed out, while the outcomes from the group practices (especially those of the Albany Practice) were scrutinised endlessly, at no point was any comparison made with any hospital cases.

An emergency meeting was called between the Albany midwives, Cathy Warwick, and Mike Savvas, Clinical Director, on 18 August 2003 to discuss the safety of the home birth service and the care provided by the Albany midwives. Mike Savvas reported that there had been concerns expressed by some of the obstetricians that the midwives were booking women for home births inappropriately and that they were not always following King's guidelines. However, as Zoe remarked, some of the neonatologists and obstetricians 'thought anybody having a home birth was crazy'. Interestingly, although there was an assumption that it was the babies born at home that were most likely to have problems, the babies on 'the list' had often been born in hospital with obstetricians supervising.

The midwives also explained that on occasion women made decisions outside the hospital guidelines, which they as midwives were required to support. The obstetricians' apparent misunderstanding about informed consent and women's decision-making became a persistent theme during later investigations. It was agreed that more open communication was needed between the midwives and the medical staff. Cathy continued to liaise with Tony Davies to make sure that any cases he was concerned about were carefully assessed ('risk managed'), and that a full explanation was provided about what had happened and why.

It is clear that in her position as Head of Midwifery and Director of Midwifery Services, Cathy was able to support and protect the Practice. Nonetheless, tensions continued to build until one of the Albany midwives finally wrote to Cathy in mid-September 2003 about an interaction with Mike Marsh, in which she had felt disrespected and 'worried that if we (the Practice) are not able to work together with him, that it could affect the care the women received'.

By the end of September 2003 relationships had further deteriorated to the point that Pauline Armstrong, the practice manager, wrote separately to Mike Marsh and to Cathy Warwick on behalf of the Practice. The midwives felt that Mike Marsh had been 'badmouthing' them with no justification and in her letter to him Pauline expressed their collective concern that communication was poor, that the midwives did not feel they were treated as equal partners in the women's care, and that ultimately, 'poor inter-professional communication places women and their babies at risk of sub-optimal care'. In her letter to Cathy, Pauline wrote that she was making a formal complaint against Mike Marsh on behalf of the Practice because 'he appears to be harassing the Practice by deliberately looking for cases that he disapproves of in order to bring us into disrepute. This week he used the expression "another one to add to the list" in relation to [a woman] who had a home birth that he disapproved of'.

While the midwives were well aware of the tensions between midwifery and medical perspectives on birth, they had little way of knowing that the increasing focus on risk management, and the financial pressures on the NHS and thus on the Trusts as the NHS was gradually prepared for privatisation, eventually combined to create a toxic culture in which a self-managed, self-employed midwifery group practice was particularly vulnerable.

These changes in the culture of maternity care and staff shortages, particularly in London, were beginning to bite. By 2003, midwifery and medical staff shortages were acute. The issue had been raised in January in the House of Lords debate, with Lord Chan commenting that 'nine out of 10 maternity units in the NHS in England have unfilled posts for midwives, and the overall and long-term vacancy rates are the highest that the Royal College of Midwives has recorded', and that 'London has critically high levels of midwife vacancies'. Baroness Perry raised similar concerns about obstetric services due to the Government having reduced 'the number of consultants in obstetrics training in 1998–99', and thus the number of training places, without considering the impact of the forthcoming European Working Time Directive.

Risk management and pressures on staff were undoubtedly two major factors in how this story unfolded. Cathy remarked that while the Clinical Director was supportive, he was anxious about maternity services in particular. There was increasing pressure on Trusts to report and justify their actions, risk managers were appointed and the risk manager in maternity at King's 'had piles of cases she was always looking at'. But Cathy stressed that this impacted on all the midwifery group practices and not just the Albany Practice.

Because of the continual questioning about the Albany Practice and other community practices by the two obstetricians and some of the neonatal staff, Cathy said she repeatedly scrutinised herself and any possible 'blindness' she might have had to seeing real problems, but for all the scrutiny and reviews she and others carried out, 'everything told me there wasn't a problem'.

Looking back over the years when Cathy Warwick was in charge of midwifery care at King's, it is clear that her approach to management was pivotal in maintaining an open and honest dialogue between the Albany Practice and the hospital staff. Her pragmatic and supportive approach both protected the Practice and addressed the concerns of the medical staff. Angela Helleur, the Local Supervising Authority Midwifery Officer at the time, described her as providing 'stalwart support' for the AMP. It was also Jane Sandall's view that by dealing with matters openly as they arose 'Cathy was the person who squared the circle and kept the whole show on the road.' Cathy Walton, in her subsequent role as a Consultant Midwife, worked closely with Cathy Warwick, and agreed that she not only worked well with the obstetricians, but also with the neonatologists: 'she just had a way about her of managing to deal with those people without getting their backs up but also being able to be firm'. Lesley Page also commented: 'Cathy's style of leadership is very sophisticated and very ethical, and I think that probably people felt very safe with her'. Cathy's insistence on a culture of 'sit down and talk' allowed for constructive discussion. Each time a challenge arose, she was able to deal with it positively. With this approach, the tensions in 2003 were finally navigated successfully, and the ongoing difficulties appeared to come to an end when Mike Marsh's role of link obstetrician for the Albany Practice was taken over by the newly appointed consultant obstetrician Leonie Penna.

Leonie taking on the role of link obstetrician occurred almost by chance. In early 2004 Becky happened to be in the labour ward office when Leonie called in to introduce herself to the labour ward staff. Becky engaged her in conversation, and took the opportunity to tell her about the Albany Practice. Leonie appeared extremely interested, and because of the recent situation with Mike Marsh, and Leonie's openness and approachability, Becky asked her almost in passing if she would consider becoming the Practice's link obstetrician. Leonie replied that she would, and very quickly took on the role. She proved to be friendly, supportive and approachable, and the tensions of the previous months appeared to settle. Indeed, when an adverse incident occurred around this time involving an Albany baby, the midwife was praised for her skilled care and her immediate and appropriate response to the situation by Professor Anne Greenough, the Director of the Children Nationwide Regional Neonatal Intensive Care Centre. Anne wrote to Cathy Warwick asking her to pass on her thanks: 'I would be grateful if you would let all the Albany Practice midwives be aware that I am very grateful for their input into the care of families we jointly look after.'

Until 2008, common sense appeared to prevail, and the unfounded negative views remained reasonably contained. However, beneath the surface these views about the model of care continued to simmer. Yet as late as 2007 King's appeared to be celebrating the Practice, and preparations for a party to celebrate the AMP were under way.

Beverley Lawrence Beech
Former Chair of AIMS and author of Am I Allowed?

When I first heard about the Albany Midwifery Practice I was so thrilled that at last we would have a system, supported by the NHS, which would enable midwives properly to practise midwifery and facilitate women's informed decision-making.

So it came as a horrible shock when I was informed that the Albany Practice was being investigated and was under threat of closure, and was shortly afterwards summarily closed down. As is often the case, it seems that the midwives involved had been told not to discuss what was happening, which meant that rumours were flying around. I and other members of the

Albany Action Group spent some considerable time trying to understand the reasons for the closure, and questioning the flawed statistics that had been used by King's to justify this.

I was outraged that such an underhand, devious action could be taken without any accountability. It further infuriated me that the newly appointed Head of Midwifery was not willing to fight for her midwives.

However, what disturbs me most is that King's was able to select the period of statistical relevance, and only examine a small number of Albany cases where the babies had poor outcomes at birth, as well as failing to compare the Albany outcomes with outcomes for King's as a whole. This made the Albany Midwifery Practice look dangerous when subsequent analysis revealed that this was clearly not the case.

Instead the analysis showed that this Practice had superb outcomes in comparison to the local obstetric units. Yet there was and still is no mechanism for reinstatement of the Practice. It seems the power to make decisions about maternity services rests entirely with the Trust, which will not acknowledge that its behaviour was unacceptable and dishonest.

The Albany Midwifery Practice had long been acknowledged as a centre of excellence. King's claimed that it closed the Practice because it had the safety of the mothers and babies at heart. In reality, by closing the Albany, King's College Hospital put women and babies at increased risk. The Albany midwives provided safe, woman-centred care for women from deeply disadvantaged backgrounds for more than 12 years. It was unacceptable and unethical to withdraw such a safe and needed service from the poorest women in society.

7
Celebrating 10 years

The groundbreaking contract between King's and the Albany Midwifery Practice had been signed in April 1997, and some time in the spring of 2007 it was decided to hold a party to celebrate 10 years of the AMP. King's was also celebrating the Practice, and a media release in July, just before the party, was headed:

> *'LONDON HOSPITAL LEADING MIDWIFERY REVOLUTION CELEBRATES 10-YEAR MILESTONE'*

The Albany midwives were good at parties. Every Christmas they invited all the women whose babies had been born in the preceding year to a party at the Practice, where they could meet up and renew acquaintance with others they had met at the antenatal or postnatal

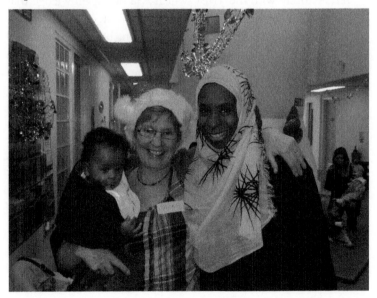

Claire and her baby with Becky at an Albany Christmas party

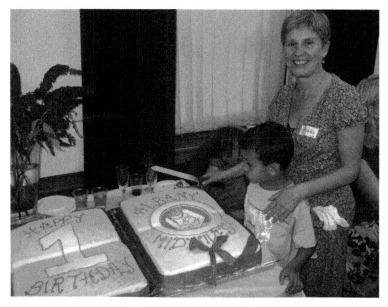

The 10-year anniversary cake

groups. These get-togethers were always wonderful occasions, with food and drink, cuddling of babies and sharing of stories.

In order to acknowledge the importance of their link with King's, the midwives decided to hold their celebration party in the board room at the hospital. A list of guests was drawn up, which included all those who had been involved with the AMP over the years, from Baroness Julia Cumberlege (author of *Changing Childbirth*) to women who had received care from the Albany midwives. A few of those women were also asked to speak, telling the story of their midwifery care. Balloons with the Albany logo were ordered, and one of the women offered to make a giant cake to share.

The board room at King's was a perfect size for the planned event, but it is a sombre room hung with large, dark paintings of stuffy-looking men in suits. The midwives decided they would prefer not to have these men looking down on them at their celebration, so they ordered poster-sized photos of women and babies who had been cared for by the Practice and used these to

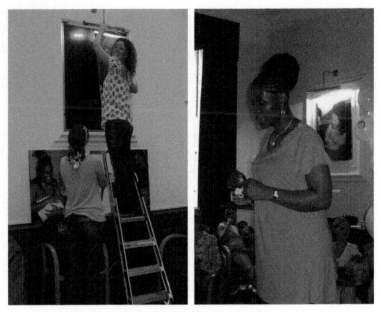

Left: *Danielle covering the paintings in the King's board room
with Albany posters* Right: *Faith talking about her care*

cover the framed pictures, as well as putting together a slideshow
of photos from the Practice to run during the speeches.

The party, in July, was a huge success – a wonderful celebration
of the first 10 years of this gold-standard midwifery practice.
Two of the women shared, very movingly, the stories of their
care. Cathy Warwick and Leonie Penna both gave very positive
speeches. Becky welcomed everyone with some thank yous, a brief
recap about the history of the Practice, and a short reminder about
why the Practice was so very special. She quoted from *Changing
Childbirth*:

> '[Women] want a service that is flexible and responsive to their
> individual needs, which acknowledges the role of their partners
> and which communicates effectively. They want improved
> information that allows them to make informed choices. Above all,
> women and their partners are seeking a service that is respectful,

personalised and kind, which gives them control and makes them feel comfortable in the sense of being at ease in the environment of childbirth and having confidence in their care.'

She went on to talk about how the Albany Practice had tried to address these goals over the previous 10 years:

'We have based ourselves in the community so that we are as accessible as possible to the women we look after. We have provided quite remarkable continuity of carer, with 97% of women having one or both of their named midwives at their birth. We have offered all healthy women with normal pregnancies real choice in where they have their babies, resulting in nearly half of the women we look after having their babies at home. Our statistics for last year (2006) are representative of this: 46% home births, 82% normal births, only 15% CS. (This is at a time when the national rate for home birth is around 2%, and CS rates are somewhere in the mid 20%). We work hard to encourage everyone to breastfeed (as you all know!), and last year 79% of mothers were exclusively breastfeeding at 28 days. We believe passionately in helping women to have normal births – this obviously includes supporting women to believe they can do this thing that after all they are designed to do...'*

Becky concluded her talk by putting those statistics into context, reminding those present why statistics matter:

'Statistics are important, and they are important because they mean something. Each woman who feels happy about her pregnancy and birth, and feels proud about what she has achieved, takes that feeling with her as she learns to be a mother. None of us who have had babies ever forgets that experience; it stays with us all our lives. As midwives we must never, ever forget this – we must always, always remember how special each birth is; it is after all the only birth for that very special baby. In this increasingly* *technological age, we must continue to believe that it matters how babies come into the world, and how their mothers – and the rest of the family – feel about their birth.'*

Cathy Warwick then spoke about the origins of the Practice and about the positive contribution to midwifery that the Albany had 'given us both at King's and nationally'.

In the light of subsequent events Leonie Penna's speech to this celebration gathering was very interesting indeed. Her speech was recorded on video:

'I have gradually learned, and I would stress how much I have learned, as a doctor and a relatively senior clinician, from the Albany midwives. I think what the Albany team brings into the hospital is this cooperation between midwives and doctors, and particularly being the advocate for the woman in a situation where perhaps doctors have a very set way of doing things. So they bring to me a situation where I'll say something should be done in a particular way, and the number of times they'll say to me "But why does it have to be done?", and when I think about it I realise it is a dogma based on very little evidence. And I think they're remarkable for the fact that they're prepared to do that because they never stop thinking about at any point in a woman's pregnancy or labour, what is the best thing for her. So it's never about what's easy for them, it's always about what's best for the woman. As Cathy [Warwick] said, there can be challenges, and I deal with challenges particularly with junior doctors where there are conflicts between them, and I think, I hope, that in the future we will actually reach a stage where all the doctors will see it as I do, which is that they have a huge amount to bring to King's and particularly to bring to the women that they look after... I want to say to you all if you have a glass let's raise our glasses to the Albany team and may they keep on [what they're doing] for a long time.'

Seventeen months later Leonie Penna was one of those accusing the Albany midwives of dangerous practice, based on a Case Series whose starting date had apparently been sixteen months *before* this positive, affirming speech. No wonder that the following year the midwives began to think they were living in a parallel universe.

On the day though there was champagne and merriment and congratulations. A few days later a letter arrived from Baroness Cumberlege:

> *'What a fabulous party. The Board Room will never have seen anything like that – stuffy old men hiding behind breastfeeding women – fabulous. The balloons were wonderful, the babies enchanting, the mothers radiant and the midwives... inspiring.*
> *Thank you for all you said about* Changing Childbirth *– if it has kept the Albany Practice alive and well it has achieved so much...*
> *See you on your 21st* [birthday].
> *With love and best wishes*
> *Julia'*

Caroline Homer
Emeritus Professor of Midwifery, University of Technology Sydney

The Albany Practice has always been a beacon of hope and an example of what is possible in the provision of midwifery continuity of care. I have followed the development of the Practice over many years and always loved hearing about the way the model of care operated. In Australia, we have used so many examples from the Albany Practice in the development of our midwifery models of care, including the antenatal groups, being based in the community, and supporting home birth as a real option. When there was an opportunity to assist in reporting the outcomes I jumped at the chance as I felt this was such an important story to tell. Analysing the data from the practice was such a privilege and I am so pleased that the paper is now out there for others to use (see Chapter 19).

When the Albany was closed I was devastated. This seemed such a travesty and I felt for the women and their families who would miss out on this way of receiving maternity care.

The Albany Practice has inspired so many models of midwifery care around the world and even though it was closed, its legacy still lives on. The Practice showed how midwifery could be provided, especially the commitment towards providing for those women with the least advantages – the population who should be our priority always but very often are not. Albany showed that continuity could be provided and midwives could work in this way – and liked working in this way. Albany showed that excellent outcomes are possible, even in communities that face multiple challenges.

I still see the Albany Practice as an exemplar of quality midwifery practice and the vision and way of working still inspires me in my work and in my commitment and determination to upscale midwifery continuity of care to all women in all countries.

8
The questions continue

At the start of 2009 the midwives and their Practice manager were feeling as though they were living in some kind of incomprehensible nightmare. They were being told that their practice was dangerous and that they were causing harm to some of the babies in their care. However, they felt that the statistics used to back up this claim were, as they described in their briefing paper to the Deputy Chief Executive, 'incomplete, inaccurate, miscalculated and subjective'.

The allegations against the midwives had been made in early December 2008, yet more than a month later there had still been no opportunity to discuss the situation with the people who were accusing them. Pauline had sent a list of questions to Katie Yiannouzis before Christmas, to provide the basis for agenda items for a meeting with Katie and Leonie to be held in January. These included questions about the way the data had been collected and analysed, and concern over the time period used. There was increasing disquiet not only about the data set itself, but also about the fact that by mid-January not one but two revisions of the original version had appeared (see Chapter 9). Added to Pauline's earlier questions were the following:

> 'We would like to talk about the process and apparent lack of transparency: why was the first meeting called in such a way?
> On what basis are the special measures we are being asked to comply with being instituted?
> Working together through this process, what now?'

On 15 January Katie and Leonie came to the Practice for a meeting with the midwives, Pauline, and Francine from the RCM. Comprehensive notes of the meeting were taken by Pauline. Francine opened with an overview of 'what we are hoping to achieve: discuss collaborative working in a non-defensive manner'.

Since the Case Series was the basis for the allegations and subsequent actions against the midwives, the discussion started with an explanation by Katie of how the data collection had come about. It appeared that throughout the maternity service there had been a series of 'red' (very serious) incidents which had been reported to the Strategic Health Authority (SHA), a body responsible for managing performance and implementing health policy at a regional level within the NHS. These organisations ceased to exist in 2013. The SHA had apparently 'got worried and started asking questions', and had suggested an external review. Leonie explained that 'the risk management database started at this point'.

It is unclear exactly when these red incidents took place, and whether or not they had anything to do with the Albany midwives. The midwives had not been made aware of the SHA's involvement at the time, nor that an external review had been suggested. Katie went on to say that 'the data source used to collate the data [the Case Series] presented to the AMP is [from] the risk management database', which Leonie felt showed a 'significantly worrying number of Albany cases of HIE'.

It was agreed that the term HIE was not easy to define (see chapters 9 and 12). Leonie suggested replacing HIE with 'term babies with unexpected and serious admissions to SCBU'. She revealed that yet another database had recently been set up 'to make definitions clearer'. It seemed to the midwives that there was a certain amount of confusion over which data were being collected, and Becky commented that 'the inference was that there is something Albany is doing to cause these babies problems.'

As has been noted before, it was becoming even clearer that some at King's believed that the Albany midwives were responsible for causing untoward outcomes in some births. It seems that this belief had become so entrenched that it was impossible to challenge, and had led to a process that had become unstoppable. As Pauline later commented:

'I think the way they did it and the statistics that they were using, the information they were using, was always unrealistic and unhelpful, so they were making these accusations, but actually, had no good evidence for it at all. But it almost seemed like, once they'd decided it was us, they were gonna make it fit.'

Leonie conceded that the measures that had been put in place might not prove to be useful. But she then stated that the AMP 'must be doing something, knowingly or unknowingly. There is a high probability that the issue resides with the Albany, though it may just turn out to be coincidence', to which Becky replied 'It is the inference of causality that has troubled us from the beginning.'

Becky had been doing some research into HIE and its incidence. When Leonie commented that the incidence of HIE following home births was 'particularly high', Becky felt confident to respond:

'Of the four cited home births [in the Case Series] two were not HIE, which would then give the AMP an expected rate of HIE incidences. We don't believe the number to be statistically significant.'

The midwives queried again how the concerns about their practice had been managed. Katie responded: 'Would you have preferred us to go ahead without letting you know?', and then said: 'We accept that you don't like the way it was done and that the statistics were messy.'

Later in the meeting came the shocking admission from Leonie that, from the time span of two years and seven months used in the Case Series, there were 17 months of data missing. The midwives and Pauline could hardly believe what they were hearing. In reply to their questioning, Leonie responded that the numbers used to show that there were many more Albany term babies admitted to SCBU with HIE compared to other King's babies were 'extrapolated'. Did this mean that the percentage of Albany babies admitted to special care compared to other King's babies was a guesstimate based on the 14 months and one day for which data were apparently available? Despite requesting clarification about this, it proved impossible to find out what Leonie meant, which data were missing, why they were missing, and how figures could possibly have been 'extrapolated'. The midwives were told that if they wanted to check this they would have to go through the SCBU data themselves. It seemed that an earlier prediction by Kate Brintworth, that the midwives might have to carry out their own research, was proving to be true.

Mary Newburn
Independent maternity consultant and service user researcher

The Albany Practice was so special; so exciting. It was that rare thing that existed in practice in the way it was dreamed of being. The offer: responsive, relationship-based, respectful midwifery care, on the NHS, provided for women and families in an inner-city area with high levels of ethnic diversity and considerable economic deprivation. Opportunities for planned home birth as a mainstream care option.

The Albany midwives provided women and families with the whole deal. Care in their homes and in their local community, care from individuals. A person with a known face and personality. Someone to see as the weeks of pregnancy passed and the birth came nearer. Someone who had become a friend and safe person to confide in, to laugh with and weep beside, by the time the baby came. So that when you were really needing a friend, you had one.

For some it is navigating the system that is the stress. The Albany was sisterhood personified. Midwives who were with women. There to empathise and understand; to inform and guide. To respect preferences and decisions. To help women and their partners realise their vision of a better birth, a safe and respectful birth, not a 'following the guidelines' birth or a 'computer-says' birth.

The Albany was there for women, for couples, for babies, for families. It had a strong committed following in the local community who took to the streets with pushchairs and placards, babies and balloons, to demonstrate support for the Albany midwives and their need for this kind of care. So what went wrong? This book is about what happened.

The criticism was that care was unsafe, evidenced by preventable cases of babies with poor outcomes. But the investigation that was commissioned was riddled with weaknesses. Miranda Scanlon (then Dodwell) and I wrote a reaction to the review, as did several others. It felt like a witch hunt. Two world-views had certainly clashed: the prevailing mainstream medical model and the 'outsider' biopsychosocial model.

The loss of the Albany was momentous for the families affected and the local community. It was devastating for the midwives who had invested so much and created something unique within the NHS, important for learning and innovation. And for maternity charities and influencers it was a shocking setback.

Ten years on, NHS England and Improvement is attempting to ensure that all women can experience maternity safety, continuity of midwifery care and carer and personalised care, all of which require adequate midwifery staffing. As a 2021 report from the Government's Health and Social Care Committee Expert Panel attests, there is an urgent need to address 'persistent health inequalities and negative birthing experiences for women from minority ethnic and socio-economically deprived backgrounds'.

The loss of the Albany may have set back this cause by decades, but personalised care and continuity of carer especially for those most in need, within a safe service, remains the order of the day.

9

'Messy' statistics

'It is wrong always, everywhere, and for anyone, to believe anything upon insufficient evidence.' William Kingdon Clifford

The closure of the Albany Midwifery Practice was based on the Trust's claim that the AMP was 'unsafe'. The statement posted on the Trust's website on 15 December 2009 asserted that 'King's College Hospital puts patient safety before all other considerations. For this reason we have terminated our contract with the Albany Midwifery Practice'. Allegations about the lack of patient safety were the only grounds that could have been used to close the service down with immediate effect without having to consult the public. Given the popularity of the Albany midwives in the local community, this would have been a difficult and time-

'King's College Hospital puts patient safety before all other considerations. For this reason we have terminated our contract with the Albany Midwives practice.
We have become concerned about the safety record of the practice in comparison with the Trust's overall maternity safety record. Our records show that whilst Albany delivered babies for 4% of all King's births, those births accounted for 42% of our full term babies born with Hypoxic Ischaemic Encephalopathy, a condition whereby brain damage may be caused by a lack of oxygen to the brain, at or around the time of delivery.
The Trust formed the view based on this evidence that babies delivered by an Albany midwife were at higher risk of contracting serious Hypoxic Ischaemic Encephalopathy (HIE)'

Statement on King's' website, December 2009

consuming exercise. So the closure relied on King's' claims that its statistics provided reliable evidence that the Practice was unsafe. These 'reliable' statistics had been described by Katie Yiannouzis as 'messy'.

An enormous amount of time and effort was expended by King's in trying to maintain its assertion that Albany term babies were experiencing more health problems at birth than other term babies born under the care of King's. The Albany midwives and their supporters, with comparatively few resources, focused their attention on highlighting concerns about the robustness of the data and trying to understand what, if anything, the Case Series actually showed.

Concerns examined in this chapter fall into four broad areas:

1. The lack of robustness and reliability of the data due to inaccuracies, poor definitions and selection bias (cherry-picking).
2. The lack of any reliable denominator. In other words, there was no total number of babies on which to base any comparison between Albany term babies born in unexpectedly poor condition and similar King's babies.
3. The lack of any relevant context, such as the mortality rates of babies and the demographics of the women.
4. The unsupported assumptions or inferences made by King's that the care given by the Albany Midwifery Practice was the cause of poor outcomes among Albany term babies.

Version one of the Case Series had been presented to the Albany midwives on 3 December 2008. It was at that very first meeting with the midwives that obstetrician Leonie Penna had pointed her finger at Becky while alleging that the AMP was responsible for 75 per cent of all term babies with HIE admitted to SCBU. The implication was that the midwives' care was dangerous.

King's College Hospital NHS Foundation Trust — Women & Children's Division 1st Dec 08

TERM BABIES BORN IN VERY POOR CONDITION

Serious risk management investigations undertaken for term babies born in unexpectedly poor condition. Cases investigated since 31st March 2006				
	Total	Hospital/other	Of total	Albany	Of total
Number of cases	37	21	57%	16	43%
HIE babies	16 *17*	4 *7*	25% *44%*	12 *10*	75% *59%*
Babies who died	10	8	80%	2	20%
Babies who are doing well	11	9	82%	2	18%
Infection	13	8	61%	5	39%

*Version 1 of the Case Series (front page) with
Albany midwives' comments and corrections*

Alarm bells had started to ring for the midwives when they added up the figures listed in the first version of the Case Series and discovered basic mistakes in the arithmetic. Becky remembers sitting at home, on the floor of her living room, staring at the front page and suddenly realising that the number of babies allegedly with HIE had been added up incorrectly. This meant that the totals and percentages included in the Case Series were incorrect. Someone at King's must have also pointed out these inaccuracies, as a revised version of the Case Series was compiled on 8 December 2008, just five days later. This second version, however, wasn't shown to the midwives until 6 January 2009, and then only unofficially by a concerned King's employee.

Unbelievably, the numbers in the second version of the Case Series *still* didn't add up correctly and a third version was produced, which was given to the midwives at the meeting with Jacqueline Docherty, Deputy Chief Executive, on 14 January 2009. This third version was simply dated January 2009 and still contained arithmetical errors.

King's College Hospital NHS Foundation Trust — Women & Children's Division 8th Dec 08

Serious risk management investigations undertaken for term babies transferred to the Neonatal Unit in unexpectedly poor condition. Cases investigated since 31st March 2006 until 31st October 2008				
	Total	Hospital/other	Of total	Albany	Of total
Number of cases	45	29	64%	16	36%
HIE babies	18 *20*	7 *10*	37% *50%*	12 *10*	63% *50%*
Babies who died	11	9	82%	2	18%
Babies who are doing well	13	11	82%	2	18%

Version 2 of the Case Series (front page)

That the first version had to be corrected twice and still contained errors hardly inspired confidence in the Trust's ability to collect and analyse data. Nor did it lead to any degree of confidence in King's inferences about the Albany midwives' care. But the conclusions drawn from the Case Series were much more concerning than numbers simply not adding up.

King's College Hospital NHS Foundation Trust			Women & Children's Division Jan 09		
Serious risk management investigations undertaken for term babies transferred to the Neonatal Unit in unexpectedly poor condition. Cases investigated since 31st March 2006 until 31st October 2008					
	Total	Hospital/other	Of total	Albany	Of total
Number of cases	45	29	65%	16	35%
HIE babies	22	11	50%	10	50%
Babies who died	11	9	82%	2	18%

Version 3 of the Case Series (front page)

The midwives were not the only ones to be concerned about the Case Series. Within five days of the meeting on 3 December, clearly troubled about the reliability of the document and how it was being used, Cathy Walton and Jill Demilew, the two Consultant Midwives, wrote to Katie Yiannouzis with a list of concerns. They noted that there was no clear definition of what was being looked at or measured, and that how this was recorded changed over the three versions. They pointed out that there was no denominator with which to compare the outcomes of Albany babies with other babies born at King's, making it difficult to draw any conclusions. Finally, they highlighted that there was no consideration of health and social factors that might have led to some Albany babies having poorer outcomes. Cathy recalled that she and Jill felt that the way that the data had been collected and presented 'was a completely inappropriate way to do it. And that's why we went to Sarah Dawson so many times, and really tried to say, "You know, you need to get someone who really knows how to put this kind of stuff together in a way that isn't so arbitrary."'

On 7 January 2009, Kate Brintworth wrote to Linda Sherratt, the Midwifery Risk Manager at King's, expressing grave doubts about the accuracy of the data and requesting that it be rechecked. She urged that no further action, or attempts to draw conclusions, should take place until the veracity of the data could be confirmed or refuted:

> 'Dear Linda
>
> I am writing to you from the perspective of being supervisory support to a number of the Albany Midwives. I understand that you have undertaken a lot of work to compile the list of babies about whom there are significant concerns. However it would be helpful for the group if you could very clearly explain the processes that you have undertaken to reach the conclusive list.
>
> This would include:
>
> How you ascertained the total number of babies admitted to SCBU (Special Care Baby Unit) in this period.
>
> How you ascertained that you were certain you had all babies who were transferred in poor condition to SCBU.
>
> What were your criteria for 'unexpectedly poor condition'?
>
> How were you sure of the completeness? What cross checking did you undertake to be certain that you had a complete data set?
>
> Whether there were any exclusions eg Ruskin women or their babies [Ruskin was a team specialising in looking after 'high risk' women]
>
> Whether you had babies who were borderline cases that were either included or excluded.
>
> I understand that this has been a huge piece of work for you and I am asking you simply because for the midwives involved it is important to them that they are clear that there is no ambiguity about this data set, as the conclusions that may be drawn from the data are profound.
>
> Thank you for responding to this in the spirit of fair enquiry.
>
> Kate'

There was no reply from Linda. Kate said: 'I never got any response to that...I don't remember ever receiving any response to it at all, either verbally or in writing, any acknowledgement of even receipt of it...'. She sent a follow up email asking for a reply and said she was 'completely blanked'.

After they were presented with the Case Series, the Albany midwives had contacted Jane Sandall for an expert opinion. She had replied saying that in her view the Case Series was flawed, and sent a document explaining how maternity data could and should be collected. She pointed out that without comparing a range of outcomes (including mortality rates) from the Albany midwives with outcomes from either King's hospital or the community midwives, any data would be meaningless. In an interview later, she stated:

> *'If you are an organisation that has concerns about perinatal safety, you should do an audit that looks at all pre-specified and predefined outcomes, which should include perinatal death. By just looking at HIE, you don't have the whole picture. We know that the Albany population is at higher socio-demographic risk than the rest of the KCH population in terms of social deprivation and ethnicity. It is possible that these babies may have died if they had been looked after by another part of KCH, but have ended up with HIE instead. We just don't know because deaths have been excluded.'*

Jane explained that it is good practice to keep records of all outcomes as they occur. Having carried out a great deal of research on safety herself, she added:

> *'If you're going to compare outcomes coming from one type of care, you have to compare like with like. People have different perceptions, so you have to do it properly. And it is not rocket science — you just follow them through and collect the information on all the outcomes... That was never done. You know, it's a bit like saying, "Midwives were burnt out because they're doing caseloading or continuity." And my response is, "Well, have you compared it with burnout levels of midwives working in other ways?" You know, if you're not comparing like with like [...].'*

As statisticians and others studied the Case Series more closely, concerns deepened. All those who were presented with the data commented on the time period chosen. The Practice had had its contract with King's for more than 11 years, but the Case Series covered a period of 31 months and one day. Alison Macfarlane, statistician and Professor of Perinatal Health at City University, London, pointed out:

> 'This is not long enough to allow the possibility for time trends to be investigated. If the compilation of the lists was prompted by concern that morbidity might be rising, then a longer series of data should have been compiled.'

It was also suggested by some commentators that the time period and therefore incomplete evidence represented an element of selection bias or 'cherry-picking' that had been used to portray the Albany Midwifery Practice outcomes in the worst possible light. Amy Brown, in her book *Informed is best*,* described this as 'choosing what you want and ignoring the rest'. As well as drawing attention to the strange time period chosen, all those critiquing the Case Series commented that King's' definitions lacked precision. The Series purported to be looking at 'term babies born in very poor condition' (first version of the Case Series) or 'term babies [...] in unexpectedly poor condition' (versions two and three), but there was never any clear definition of what 'unexpectedly poor condition' meant and on what basis babies would be included or excluded from the data. Even the definition 'term' was not adhered to: the Series included an Albany baby who was born before 37 weeks and would therefore have been classed as preterm rather than term. Also included was an Albany term baby who was born in very good condition but became ill on the King's postnatal ward two days later under the care of

---

* *Informed is best: How to spot fake news about your pregnancy, birth and baby* (Pinter & Martin, 2019)

the hospital staff. Other terminology was equally imprecise. The 'outcomes' column, for example, sometimes included a diagnosis rather than an outcome, or even a subjective description, such as a baby 'doing well'.

One of the most serious problems of definition was the term 'HIE'. As Alison Macfarlane commented, 'The definition of "HIE" is a major problem. A report by NPEU [National Perinatal Epidemiology Unit]* identified 11 different definitions...'. She suggested that King's should have specified which definition it was using.

Even more seriously, statisticians and others were as concerned as the midwives about the assumption that the apparently high rate of HIE among Albany term babies was caused by poor midwifery care during labour. Alison Macfarlane commented on this in an email to the midwives about the Case Series, saying that the report from the NPEU mentioned above confirmed that: 'in many but an unknown proportion of babies, problems arose before labour'. HIE was being redefined as neonatal encephalopathy (NE) to reflect this understanding and to remove the potential for blaming practitioners. It is of course possible for poor care during labour and birth to result in HIE / NE, but this is relatively rare, as noted by Denis Walsh:

> 'Concerns were expressed about the Albany Group's prevalence of Hypoxic ischaemic encephalopathy (HIE) on the basis of their intrapartum care though it is well known that HIE is overwhelmingly related to antenatal causation and assigning causation to intrapartum events is highly problematic. Because this link is so rare, it would be nigh impossible to make judgements about the Albany Group's rate compared with the hospital's rate, unless they had accumulated tens of thousands of births'.

---

* National Perinatal Epidemiology Unit. Reaching consensus on the definition of neonatal encephalopathy for surveillance purposes. www.npeu.ox.ac.uk/ topics/project/1.1.1 Accessed November 5 2009.

It is surprising that a prestigious teaching hospital was not more aware of the complexities of diagnosing HIE, and not more cautious about drawing any inferences about the care provided.

Alison Macfarlane additionally noted that no follow-up of the babies was mentioned, despite recommendations in the medical literature that babies thought to have suffered from HIE or NE should be followed up for two years. Because of their ongoing relationships with many of the families they cared for, the midwives were aware that at least one of the Albany babies diagnosed with HIE and included in the Case Series made a complete recovery.

Further concerns were expressed about the lack of relevant information provided about the Albany mothers, or about the babies diagnosed by King's with HIE at birth. The NPEU had already published work showing that male babies – especially those born to older and younger mothers – are more likely to be affected by NE, but the Case Series included nothing about the sex of the babies or the age of the mothers. Nor was there any mention that disadvantaged women are more likely to lose their babies or have babies with health problems. A reliable account of the data would have considered the demographic and other relevant differences between Albany mothers and babies and other King's women and babies, and would have adjusted the data to reflect this.

Alison Macfarlane summarised the various concerns about the Case Series and explained why the data did not support King's' claims that the Albany midwives were providing unsafe care. She concluded:

> 'In the absence of information about the sources of the data in these Case Series, the definitions and inclusion criteria used, the longer term outcome of the babies who survived, the extent to which the babies included and all babies delivered at King's had factors which were associated with neonatal encephalopathy and the lack of denominators and statistical power, it is impossible

to draw any inferences. The lack of definitions and inclusion criteria call into question these case series as a sampling frame for any investigations to be undertaken in greater depth.'

Despite the shortcomings highlighted by this experienced statistician and others, the process of attempting to prove the allegations against the Practice seemed unstoppable, a sentiment shared by Cathy Walton when she commented on the efforts she and Jill Demilew made to raise concerns about the validity of the three Case Series documents:

'we just felt palmed off a lot of the time really and there were obviously attempts to redraft it in various ways, weren't there? Which I can only assume was in some recognition that it actually wasn't terribly robust. But, you know, they'd sort of come that far... [there was a sense that] they've got themselves, however it happened, into that situation and had really no idea how to get out of it.'

But as Pauline pointed out, she and the midwives continued to hope and assume that the poor quality of evidence would eventually be revealed and lead to common sense prevailing:

'it never did make sense, did it? All the way through, the people they were including weren't all in the right category or they'd included somebody that shouldn't have been there and I mean, the whole thing was so poorly done that again, I think it kind of made me think, well, we're going to get through this because this is just silly. They can't possibly think they're going to take this any further. We just need to show them. We just need somebody to see a bit of sense and we'll sort it out.'

Meanwhile, with no sign of willingness from the Trust to re-examine the data it had compiled, the midwives decided to take matters into their own hands by checking the data themselves. In an email to Becky at the end of January, Katie said that the books from the Special Care Baby Unit (SCBU) were not available because they were being used for an audit. She offered to provide the midwives with a copy of the monthly sheets that were compiled by one of the consultant neonatologists to record all the term admissions of babies to the Neonatal Unit.

The monthly sheets were finally made available to the midwives in March 2009, and Becky and Zoe spent two long days at King's, in a tiny windowless room, carefully going through the data. They were interested in checking the total number of all King's unexpected term admissions to SCBU compared with the number of Albany babies in that category admitted over the 31 month and one day period. They discovered that six weeks of data were missing from the monthly sheets, although they were able to check their own records for information about Albany babies during that time. They also found that the way the SCBU data were presented was at times incorrect. For example, the column headed 'diagnosis' sometimes contained descriptive accounts of the baby's birth, such as 'meconium stained liquor', 'acute blood loss from unclamped cord' and 'water birth at home' rather than a diagnosis. It was therefore not surprising to the midwives that the Case Series had lacked clarity and precision. It seems as shocking now as it did then to see how unsystematically such important data on term babies admitted to SCBU were being collected.

As Becky and Zoe worked their way through the handwritten data for the 31 months and one day in question, it appeared that of the 502 documented unexpected term admissions to SCBU, 15 were Albany babies. Even without the missing six weeks of King's data, the midwives' calculation showed that for unexpected term admissions to SCBU, Albany babies accounted for less than 3 per cent of the total. What did this mean? While the midwives recognised that this was only descriptive data, and included all term babies admitted rather than only those diagnosed with HIE, it was nevertheless puzzling, as it seemed very different from the picture portrayed by King's in the Case Series.

At least two issues emerged from the midwives' careful examination of the monthly sheets. First of all, there appeared to be many different reasons why term babies could be admitted to SCBU, but by deciding to select babies who were described as having HIE and not looking at mortality rates, King's had introduced a bias against the Albany midwives' outcomes that appeared to confirm its belief that their care was unsafe. Secondly, Becky and Zoe found no evidence of the 'clusters' which had been mentioned by King's on several occasions. The number of Albany babies admitted each month was consistently either none or one, with two babies admitted in only three of the 31 months.

This idea that there was a 'cluster' of Albany term babies born in unexpectedly poor condition seemed to have been circulating for some time among some King's managers and senior health practitioners. However, as Ben Goldacre, physician and science writer, commented in his book *Bad Science*,* we tend to look for these and find them: 'We see patterns where there is only random noise'. In addition, without some knowledge of statistics, many people do not believe that genuine clusters can occur by chance, or that unlikely coincidences are much more common than they think. This might explain why King's managers thought they had identified a cluster of babies with HIE, and why this quickly led to the belief that there was a problem, prompting the compilation of the Case Series.

It seems inconceivable that these unchecked, out of context, 'messy' statistics formed the basis for months of monitoring of the midwives' practice, for the external review by CMACE, and for the eventual closure of the Albany Midwifery Practice.

---

* *Bad Science*, Ben Goldacre (2009), Fourth Estate

Wendy Savage

Honorary Professor, Middlesex University, Faculty of Health, Social Care and Education

In 1995 the late Marsden Wagner, Regional Officer for maternal and child health in the WHO European Region, published a hard-hitting article in the *Lancet* entitled 'A global witch hunt'. He drew on his experience of defending midwives, GPs and obstetricians in 10 countries over a 20-year period whose practice had been questioned. Some had been arrested, others suspended or barred from practice, not on the basis of evidence but because their practice did not fit the orthodox medical model. I was one of those obstetricians, and my story, which inspired a national campaign in 1985, was told in my book *A Savage Enquiry** (published the following year). Despite its good outcomes, the closure of the Albany Midwifery Practice in 2009 seems another example of the exercise of power by the medical profession against midwives who have a different approach to maternity care. There were allegations about babies admitted to the Neonatal Intensive Care Unit with avoidable brain damage over a 31-month period. These cases were referred to CMACE, but some have questioned the methodology of the CMACE approach and the validity of its criticisms based on small numbers and retrospective case note review. Professor Alison Macfarlane, an expert in health statistics, concluded in her analysis that it was 'impossible to draw any inferences' from the data presented. Having read the report myself, I noticed that it did not specify how many infants were admitted to the King's Neonatal Unit overall during the period analysed. This seems a basic piece of data in any enquiry.

The managerial approach to the problem seems unprofessional, with no attempt to involve the midwives in discussing King's' concerns at an early stage, and then closing the Practice without giving the Albany midwives a chance to respond to the CMACE Report.

---

* *A Savage Enquiry*, Wendy Savage (1986), Virago

The closure also had a wider impact. Women's choice has been restricted to the medical model, as I think midwifery managers are frightened of criticism in the light of the fate of the Albany Practice. The reports of recent scandals in various maternity units cite poor relationships between obstetricians and midwives, and criticise normal birth among other things. However, they seem to overlook the ongoing serious understaffing of midwifery services. Without sufficient midwives to provide excellent woman-centred professional care, mistakes will be made and women will fail to get the birth experience that they deserve.

The result of this high-handed action, which included referring one midwife to the midwifery disciplinary body, was that women in South London were deprived of an excellent model of midwifery care; a model that had allowed many to give birth at home and with better outcomes, lower intervention rates and higher and more prolonged breastfeeding rates.

10
The internal audit at King's

Throughout the first half of 2009, the Albany midwives continued to question the reliability of the data in the Case Series. They repeatedly requested that it be re-examined, but by May 2009 King's was still refusing to do this.

In June, however, it was agreed that an internal audit would be carried out. At a meeting on 1 June 2009, Katie informed the midwives that she would find 'someone new' to re-examine the data, and in correspondence on 5 June she confirmed that she was 'charging someone with trawling through the database'. To the midwives' and others' dismay, the 'someone new' turned out to be a senior Sister and renal project manager from the King's Clinical Effectiveness Department rather than an external, professional statistician. It became apparent that the renal nurse was merely being asked to check the data already collected, so therefore it could only confirm King's' hypothesis that Albany babies were more likely to be admitted to SCBU with HIE than other King's babies. As Ben Goldacre remarked: 'if your hypothesis comes from analysing the data then there is no sense in analysing the same data again to confirm it'. But this is what was done and was evidently deemed to be adequate by the Trust.

Whatever the outcome of the audit, it became clear that its conclusions were not going to have any impact on the CMACE investigation. Katie even admitted this at the June meeting. She also admitted once again that 'the way the percentages were calculated was not perfect'. And to the midwives' utter incredulity that the accuracy of the data seemed not to matter, she went on to say that this was 'water under the bridge now and nothing could be done about it'. The audit was far too little too late and, in the end, was finally published only two weeks before the CMACE report, in November 2009. It is difficult not to conclude that the internal audit was merely an ineffective attempt to appease the midwives and those who had repeatedly called for the data to be checked.

Once the audit was finally made available, reviews were carried out at the midwives' request by two independent statisticians, Professor Alison Macfarlane of City University, and Jane Galbraith, Honorary Senior Research Associate in the Department of Statistical Science at University College London. Alison's only prior contact with the Albany midwives was when she responded to their request to look at the Case Series. Jane had never heard of the Albany midwives or met any of them before being approached to give a view on the internal audit. Unsurprisingly, they both highlighted similar problems to those raised about the Case Series.

Both of these reviewers commented on the inappropriate time frame used for the internal audit, which remained the same as in the Case Series. They noted that the number of babies born in unexpectedly poor condition at term documented in the Case Series changed yet again in the audit. They pointed out that definitions in the audit remained as imprecise as they had in the Case Series documents, and yet again, neither 'poor outcome', nor 'HIE' were defined. They questioned why an Albany baby born at 36 weeks and 6 days was included in an audit that purported to be examining term babies. As in the Case Series, it is difficult not to conclude that the only reason to alter a well-recognised definition of 'term' was to be able to include an Albany baby who should not have been included in the Case Series, the internal audit or the CMACE investigation. Margaret Jowitt, who had previously been an NHS audit clerk, suggested that the vague definition of 'poor condition' and subsequent selection bias in the internal audit undermined King's' statement on its website that the Albany Midwifery Practice was responsible for 42 per cent of cases of HIE at King's College Hospital, and went on to remark that 'this "audit" feels more and more like a fishing expedition'.

Jane Galbraith suggested that while it might seem as though more Albany babies were referred to SCBU, an alternative explanation could be that 'the differences in figures are artefacts of the definitions and comparisons made and that, in fact, the Albany Group did not differ from the "core midwives" and the other maternity group practices in terms of risk to the babies they delivered'.

This idea of alternative explanations for the data was raised by several people for different reasons, none of which could have been either refuted or verified without further well-designed research being carried out. For example, Professor Mavis Kirkham had suggested that the continuity of care provided by the Albany midwives might well have provided an explanation for the very low mortality rates among Albany babies and the apparently higher number of term babies experiencing HIE at birth. In a communication reported in the winter 2009 issue of *Midwifery Matters* magazine, she commented:

> 'It may well be possible that out of their cases that end up in SCBU, Albany Midwives do have a higher proportion of HIE than other providers of care. They may well send fewer babies in for respiratory distress, neonatal jaundice and all the other consequences of interventionist birth. "Their" babies stay longer in utero, so there are fewer preterm births. One of the consistent findings supporting caseload midwifery is that admissions to SCBU are lower. We know that the Albany Midwives have an unusually low perinatal mortality rate. Could it be that the midwives are facilitating the live birth of already compromised babies who would not have survived obstetric delivery?'

A letter to King's from the NCT in February 2010 also suggested that demographic differences between Albany mothers and other King's mothers may have played a part: 'it is possible that babies at high risk were born alive under Albany care but had HIE whereas in another part of your service may not have survived'.

The lack of context in the Case Series remained a problem in the internal audit. Jane Galbraith commented that essential demographic information about the Albany mothers was omitted, with no information about their 'ethnic origin, age and lifestyle', which might have impacted on their babies' outcomes. Alison Macfarlane noted that there was no information about whether the demographic mix of the women varied between the Albany Midwifery Practice, the other midwifery group practices and those experiencing regular King's care. She also reiterated that no information was provided about how the babies were doing at 12 or 24 months of age. This follow-up was considered good practice at the time.

One difference between the Case Series and the internal audit was that the renal nurse who compiled the audit attempted to provide a way of comparing outcomes for Albany babies with outcomes for other King's babies, allowing for more meaningful conclusions to be drawn. Both Alison and Jane pointed out that various data were missing and that the information provided still didn't enable comparisons to be made. For example, different time periods were used when comparing outcomes for King's babies and Albany babies.

Just as in the Case Series, the most damning criticism of the audit was the inference of causality. It was based on the same incorrect assumption that the Albany babies born at term with HIE must have received poor care from the midwives. It cannot be overstated that the data produced by King's in the internal audit, like those in the Case Series, simply could not support this assumption.

Dr Denis Walsh
Retired Associate Professor in Midwifery

I first came across what was then known as the South-East London Midwifery Group Practice in 1994 while working in a Team Midwifery Project in Leicester, where we were beginning to explore the implementation of continuity of care models. Back then, I was impressed by this radical model of midwifery care that was a ground-up, small-scale local initiative with childbearing women at the centre. It challenged our top-down, professional-centric approach. Over the next 20 years, I kept abreast of their development into the Albany Midwifery Practice, their commissioning by King's College, their subsequent suspension and ultimate redemption though not reinstitution via hugely impressive outcome data sets published in recent years.

In midwifery circles there was much talk in the 1990s and beyond about woman-centred care and continuity of care models. In retrospect, I view this as a largely professional project, despite the fact the continuity element had an emerging evidence base. But midwifery had been in a territorial dispute with obstetrics over centuries and usually was the loser when it came to who exercised real power over the maternity services. It was understandable, therefore, that the profession took opportunities to exert some agency in policy and practice where it could. The Albany midwives set up their project with local women as partners and built a service tailored to their needs. I suspect that if you had told them that the emerging evidence supported such a model, they would have said common sense informed their priorities long before the research caught up. By a master stroke, their model foregrounded home birth as the default choice for normal childbirth and therefore largely protected them from institutional oversight and interference.

Eventually, as the internal market in health extended its remit to maternity care, they were commissioned by enlightened midwifery purchasers to provide care as the Albany group under the auspices of King's Healthcare Trust. In this way, their profile rose and they became a beacon of best practice in a number of ways: a radical continuity of carer model, being self-regulating and autonomous, offering place of birth choices that included the highest home birth rate in the UK, an enlightened and flexible risk assessment model that was not arbitrary but personalised to individual women and their circumstances: all premised on emerging outstanding clinical outcomes.

The history of what happened next is well documented.

For me their unsung legacy, rarely mentioned, but hugely significant for so many midwives, was their action for social and gender justice at a time when both were marginal to policy concerns. Here was a service for women, run by women, accountable to women very often near the bottom of the socio-economic ladder. My hope is that history acknowledges this contribution equally alongside the innovative aspects of their model of care.

11
Parallel universe

'I feel like I am diagonally parked in a parallel universe' Anon

Just before the AMP's 10th anniversary party in 2007, King's had issued a media release:

> 'A *midwifery practice at King's College Hospital that is changing the face of midwifery care is celebrating 10 years of successfully serving women in South East London.*
>
> *Set up in 1997, the Albany Midwifery Practice is the UK's only self employed and self managed midwifery practice and has provided the highest level of care for over 2,000 women during one of the most important times of their lives.*
>
> *Based in the Peckham Pulse Community Centre, the midwifery practice is changing the culture of birth in the inner city community it serves and is dramatically improving women's experience of pregnancy.*
>
> *The practice [...] serves an ethnically diverse community in one of the most socially deprived areas of the country and is fast becoming a model of innovation for midwifery practices across the country.'*

In 2007 there was no reason for anyone to doubt this affirmation of the Albany model of care. Indeed King's seemed proud to celebrate the AMP and its achievements. But by the end of the following year things looked very different. The first version of the Case Series was presented to the midwives in December 2008, purporting to show how dangerous they were, and the whole sorry saga leading to the closure of the Practice had been set in motion.

During 2009, while dealing with all the allegations of dangerous practice, the midwives were confused more than once by examples of 'parallel universe' thinking – situations where they felt at the

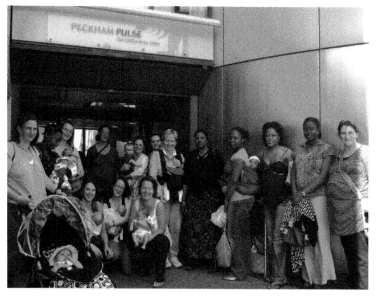

Women and babies outside Peckham Pulse, May 2007

same time both vilified and lauded.

Katie Yiannouzis, the Head of Midwifery, was supporting – outwardly at least – the Trust's efforts to condemn the Practice and prove that the midwives were practising dangerously. In early 2009 accusations were rife, the CMACE review had been commissioned, and the midwives were being subjected to monitoring of their clinical skills as well as being closely observed at their Birth Talks to check that they weren't influencing women's choices.

In early April 2009 Heather (not her real name), who was pregnant with her second baby, wrote to Katie as Head of Midwifery to ask for her support. Heather had had a traumatic first birth at King's, following which she had had a debriefing meeting with Cathy Walton in Cathy's position as Consultant Midwife. During the discussion Cathy had suggested that if Heather were to have another baby she should consider contacting Katie early on in her pregnancy, to discuss organising a plan of midwifery care. Heather had heard of the Albany and was interested in its model of continuity of carer, saying 'having one midwife through the term of my pregnancy would bring quickly to the fore any issues as and when they occurred, rather than afterwards, when it was too late.'

So at seven weeks pregnant Heather wrote to Katie asking for her assistance. This was a woman who was suffering ongoing gynaecological problems after a poor experience with her previous birth. A woman who was asking for something better. A pregnant woman searching for excellent midwifery care. The day after receiving the letter Katie emailed the AMP:

> 'Dear Albany midwives
> Could you possibly help by taking Heather – see the email below.
> Please let me know.
> Thanks
> Katie'

What was Katie thinking when she made this request? Had she momentarily forgotten that King's was questioning the Albany midwives' practice? Did she really believe that the midwives were dangerous? It was almost unthinkable that she was referring a woman who was looking for the best possible care following a previous traumatic birth, who had had every reason to complain to the Trust after her earlier experience, to the AMP. And yet, as Zoe commented later, this had become common practice within the Trust:

> 'Katie often contacted us to look after women that they basically felt no one else could look after. Because they had, you know, complicated stories or wanted things that were outside the guidelines. So it seemed very strange then to be criticised for supporting women who were making those choices, when they had often put women in touch with us just because of knowing that we would support women to make their own decisions. Which ultimately was what we were doing.'

In another strange twist, Jenny (not her real name), a local schoolgirl who was the daughter of a friend of Leonie's, emailed Leonie in March

2009 to ask for help with finding a work placement. Jenny was very specific in her email, requesting 'a placement for work shadowing in the Albany Midwifery Practice'. Leonie apparently never received this email, so Jenny wrote again a couple of weeks later, reiterating that she 'would love a placement with the Albany Team'. Leonie replied immediately, saying 'I have sent your email on to the Albany midwives and Becky will get in touch with you.' Although Leonie also offered Jenny in this email 'the option of spending some time in the maternity department at King's shadowing a hospital based midwife', this was clearly a second choice if shadowing the AMP midwives didn't work out: 'I suggest you correspond with Becky initially, and depending on what she is able to arrange we could add some KCH sessions.'

Leonie clearly had the opportunity to steer this young girl away from observing midwives whose practice she was in the process of questioning. And yet, in spite of her apparent very serious concerns, she willingly supported Jenny's work placement with these very midwives. Leonie passed Jenny's mobile number on to Becky in an email at the start of May, signing off with 'See you soon. Lx'. Jenny went on to have a very successful week in June shadowing the midwives and learning all about the Albany model of care.

Another story involved Beth (not her real name), a barrister who was expecting her first baby at the end of April 2009. Her pregnancy had continued past her due date, and Becky had taken over as her primary midwife for the birth.

In a reflection some years later, Beth wrote that her baby was born 'nearly 3 weeks over dates, and at a time when it has now become apparent that Becky and the whole Albany Practice were being assessed for alleged poor practice.' Beth was 'longing' for a home birth, and was concerned at going past her due date, as both her mother and her sister had been induced at 42 weeks of pregnancy and ended up having caesarean sections. As Beth's pregnancy continued, Becky was liaising with Leonie Penna about her care. Beth says:

> 'I remember being in the Albany office for check-ups while Becky
> liaised with King's about me coming in to meet one of the

consultant obstetricians. At no point was there ever any concern expressed by King's in the conversations that I ought to be rushed in to meet them – the impression given was that they had absolute confidence in Becky and the Albany Practice.'

A plan was made for Beth to have a consultation with Leonie at 42 weeks and 3 days, and, as was her usual practice, Becky attended the appointment with Beth. Beth says:

'The whole meeting had a very positive and light-hearted atmosphere. It felt as though Dr Penna and Becky were a team who had a great deal of mutual respect for each other. There was no hint at all that there was any concern with either Becky's professional opinion or her practice when Becky was in the room or when she was out of the room.'

Beth admits in her reflection that, being a barrister, she was 'probably approaching everything from a very analytical perspective as a consequence.' But thanks to this her analysis of the situation is astute and powerful:

'If King's had real concerns about Becky's abilities then why did they leave her to handle me at 42+3, 42+4, 42+5 etc. unsupervised in what they would have regarded as a risky situation? Why were they being so publicly supportive of her when, in their minds, her conduct was putting their patients at risk? Why were they proposing even more risky options which she might oversee [Leonie had discussed the option of breaking Beth's waters and then Beth labouring at home 'with Becky to supervise me'] if they didn't believe in her and her abilities? If King's actually held the concerns which they now claim to about Becky then they would also have believed that they were leaving myself and J [her baby] at real risk in our particular circumstances, and not only did they give absolutely no impression that that was the case, but they made no attempt whatsoever to do anything about it.'

Beth had an uncomplicated birth at home, with Becky in attendance, at nearly three weeks past her due date.

The examples above illustrate a strange scenario in the first half of 2009. It was as though there were two Albany Practices – the 'real' and the 'imagined'. In the 'real' Practice life for the midwives continued as it always had, apart from the obvious intrusions of extra monitoring of the midwives' clinical practice, and the underlying constant anxiety about what the future might hold. But the 'imagined' Practice had a much darker side, with the accusations against it of dangerous midwifery leading to damaged babies. And it genuinely seemed that the boundaries between the two had become so blurred that certain behaviours and actions didn't make sense any more.

Throughout this time other examples of parallel universe thinking were playing out. In July 2007 a report (*Healthcare for London: A Framework for Action Report*, for London boroughs' health overview and scrutiny committees) was published by Professor Sir Ara Darzi. It was commissioned in 2006 to review London's healthcare by the newly-formed NHS London, the Strategic Health Authority for London. It proposed radically new models of healthcare and how these could be provided, and included a chapter on 'Maternity and newborn care'. This specified that women should receive care from individual or small groups of midwives and envisioned a 'more effective use of midwives and the development of a new and sustainable model of service provision'. It suggested that there were already examples in London of how a 'maternity workforce can provide personalised and high-quality care...' and cited the Albany Midwifery Practice as its case study. In a follow-up report in October 2007, the Albany was again cited. In his recommendations for ongoing consultation, Sir (now Lord) Darzi suggested that:

> 'If Members decide to visit any healthcare facilities in the course of the review, they might wish to visit some of the facilities referred to in the report as providing examples of good practice, such as [...] the Albany midwife-led maternity practice.'

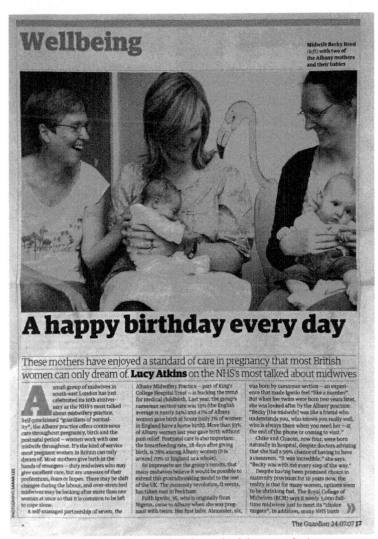

Wellbeing

Midwife Becky Reed (left) with two of the Albany mothers and their babies

A happy birthday every day

These mothers have enjoyed a standard of care in pregnancy that most British women can only dream of. **Lucy Atkins** on the NHS's most talked about midwives

A small group of midwives in south-east London has just celebrated its 10th anniversary as the NHS's most talked about midwifery practice. Self-proclaimed "guardians of normality", the Albany practice offers continuous care throughout pregnancy, birth and the postnatal period – women work with one midwife throughout. It's the kind of service most pregnant women in Britain can only dream of. Most mothers give birth in the hands of strangers – duty midwives who may give excellent care, but are unaware of their preferences, fears or hopes. There may be shift changes during the labour, and over-stretched midwives may be looking after more than one woman at once so that it is common to be left to cope alone.

A self-managed partnership of seven, the Albany Midwifery Practice – part of King's College Hospital Trust – is bucking the trend for medical childbirth. Last year, the group's caesarean section rate was 15% (the English average is nearly 24%) and 47% of Albany women gave birth at home (only 2% of women in England have a home birth). More than 93% of Albany women last year gave birth without pain relief. Postnatal care is also important: the breastfeeding rate, 28 days after giving birth, is 78% among Albany women (it is around 20% in England as a whole).

So impressive are the group's results, that many midwives believe it would be possible to extend this groundbreaking model to the rest of the UK. The maternity revolution, it seems, has taken root in Peckham.

Faith Igwilo, 36, who is originally from Nigeria, came to Albany when she was pregnant with twins. Her first baby, Alexander, six, was born by caesarean section – an experience that made Igwilo feel "like a number". But when her twins were born two years later, she was looked after by the Albany practice: "Becky [the midwife] was like a friend who understands you, who knows you really well, who is always there when you need her – at the end of the phone or coming to visit."

Chike and Chisom, now four, were born naturally in hospital, despite doctors advising that she had a 99% chance of having to have a caesarean. "It was incredible," she says. "Becky was with me every step of the way."

Despite having been promised choice in maternity provision for 10 years now, the reality is that for many women, options seem to be shrinking fast. The Royal College of Midwives (RCM) says it needs 3,000 full-time midwives just to meet its "choice targets". In addition, many NHS birth ▶▶

PHOTOGRAPHS: SARAH LEE

The Guardian 24.07.07 17

The Guardian *article 'A happy birthday every day'*

Also in July 2007, the *Guardian* newspaper ran an article about 'the NHS's most talked about midwives'. With the title 'A happy birthday every day', it described the Albany Practice and commented on the 'impressive' outcomes for the previous year, saying: 'many midwives believe it would be possible to extend this groundbreaking model to the rest of the UK'. The article emphasised the importance of continuity of care as 'the bedrock of [The Albany's] success', and quoted Jane Sandall: 'We have learned so much from Albany about improving outcomes for women and babies... This is the future of midwifery care'.

In early 2007 a research project started to take shape which was to continue until the very moment that the Albany midwives were initially made aware of the accusations against them. This research project was commissioned by the Department of Health (England) as one of six projects to support the implementation of the National Service Framework (NSF), which stated that multidisciplinary training should promote a shared philosophy of care so that 'women are supported and encouraged to have as normal a pregnancy and birth as possible, with medical interventions recommended only if they are of benefit to the woman or her baby'. The aim was to develop and field-test an 'interactive, multi-disciplinary learning package to increase midwives' and doctors' confidence and competence in supporting women to have a "normal" birth, in particular where a woman has chosen to labour without pharmacological intervention.' Because of its innovative model of working and especially because of its outstanding outcomes, the Albany Midwifery Practice was chosen as the example in the study.

In an article about the research published in 2009, the authors explained the background to the participants and settings involved in the project:

> 'A midwifery group practice in an inner city setting in England was the main setting chosen to study exemplary practice and the testimony of women who were cared for by these midwives. In spite of working in an area of high socio-economic deprivation, this community based midwifery practice has been particularly successful in facilitating normal birth, a positive experience for women and their families and improved outcomes.'

In the same article there is a strong emphasis on the importance of collaborative inter-professional working:

'In designing and developing the learning package, we recognised the importance of addressing the principles and practicalities of effective interprofessional learning in a research process that would foster the potential for midwives and medical staff to... learn with, from and about each other to improve collaboration and the quality of care.'

This huge, multi-faceted piece of work, involving interviews, video recordings and workshops, was designed to evaluate an educational tool that could be used nationwide. The final report, which ran to 182 pages, was published in June 2010 by the Health and Social Care Research Division of King's College, London, under the title *Supporting women to have a normal birth: Development and field testing of a learning package for maternity staff.* However, by the time of its publication the exemplary Albany Midwifery Practice had been closed down on grounds of 'patient safety'. The project had found that the educational tool could, and did, make a difference, but because of the investigations into the Albany Practice the findings were not pursued by the Department of Health. Jane Sandall, one of the lead authors of the report, thought the Department: 'can't be seen to be endorsing as good practice a model of care that might in the long term come out to be seen as risky'.

Dangerous or exemplary? The Albany Midwifery Practice could surely not have been both.

Sarah Davies
Retired Senior Midwifery Lecturer, Salford University

In 1990 I started work as a midwife teacher, and at some point in the early 1990s I heard Becky speak at a midwives' meeting in Manchester. I listened enthralled as she described what I considered the dream set-up for midwives and women – midwives contracted into the NHS, but self-managing and autonomous, part of their community and supporting all their women to have births that were right for them. From then on, the Albany was always in my midwifery consciousness – a beacon of hope, and an example I often used with students to explain the power and the rewards of true midwifery. We discussed how we might be able to get 'an Albany everywhere' within the NHS. Over the next decade and a half, many of my students went to spend time with the Albany midwives. They always felt welcomed and returned inspired, with a better knowledge of midwifery, some great birth stories, and a deeper understanding of the value of continuity of midwifery carer. Those experiences stayed with them once they'd qualified and several went on to set up or join continuity and home birth schemes themselves, building a network of supportive relationships in their communities.

So I was aghast when I heard that the AMP had been suddenly closed. In that moment I knew I would do whatever was in my power to support the Albany midwives. I was used to the entrenched power struggles in midwifery and the bullying of 'tall poppies' i.e. midwives who stood up for the best evidence-based care for women. I'd experienced some of it myself. But for this to happen to our gold-standard Albany practice, which had been acclaimed as an example of good practice in the UK and internationally, was utterly shocking. And I felt distressed for those women who would be deprived of their midwives when they needed them.

The campaign to Save the Albany was utterly inspiring, as was the tenacity and creativity of the Albany mums. The range and number of people and organisations who rallied to the cause was remarkable. But the Trust had decided, for whatever reason, that it didn't want the Albany any more. Those who authorised the closure acted unjustly, citing safety reasons, knowing that in doing so they could bypass the normal scrutiny procedures for such a decision. To be wrongly accused of unsafe practice is highly traumatic, but they seemed not to care about this damage to the Albany midwives, who had given years of dedicated service. I knew Albany was the safest care for families, and this was borne out by the Practice statistics when they were analysed in detail and published, long after the closure.

But the Albany model lives on, in people's minds, in academic literature, in articles and now in this book. This story is even more important today, as wholesale privatisation of the NHS looms and we will need to continue to fight for good maternity care for all women. The Albany model worked because midwives had the autonomy to use their full range of skills and to organise themselves. It worked because it was open to every woman whatever her income or 'risk status'. It is still a beacon of hope.

12

'The London Project': the CMACE review

At the very first meeting with King's in December 2008 the Albany midwives heard about the plan to commission an external review in response to the fear that this group of midwives was practising dangerously. As Kate Brintworth said:

> 'You have to remember that they believed that this was real. People were really really really concerned... If you suspend disbelief for a moment about the construction of that data [Case Series], and move to the position where you believed that the construction of that data was good, then what that was saying was really really worrying. That there is one group of midwives within the umbrella of this organisation for whom we are repeatedly seeing poor outcomes. As an organisation we can't just pretend that isn't happening.'

The Albany midwives knew that the construction of the data definitely wasn't 'good'. As Leonie Penna had admitted, the data set had been hastily put together and was 'not as polished as it could be'. But she had also said 'We do need to be seen to be doing something.' Whether or not the data were correct seemed less relevant than the institution's reputation. The thought seemed to be that King's might be deemed to be negligent if it didn't act on the apparent findings of the Case Series by putting in place a number of measures, which included the commissioning of an external review.

Investigations into maternal and infant deaths have been

carried out in England since the early 20th century. When King's commissioned the confidential enquiry into the Albany Midwifery Practice, the organisation they contacted was CEMACH (Confidential Enquiry into Child and Maternal Health), which had been set up in April 2003. CEMACH had replaced CESDI (the Confidential Enquiry into Stillbirths and Deaths in Infancy) and CEMD (the Confidential Enquiry into Maternal Deaths). The change in title was to 'better describe the enquiry's concern with morbidity as well as mortality'.

On 1 July 2009, in the middle of the Albany review, CEMACH became an independent charity. Its name was changed to CMACE (Centre for Maternal and Child Enquiries). Many people were concerned about this change in status, and noticed that this so-called 'independent' charity was accepting adverts from commercial organisations, including some involved in childbirth. It was also accepting direct commissions from healthcare Trusts, for which it was paid significant amounts of money. Both of these potential conflicts of interest could have impacted on its investigations.

The midwives felt confident that what they assumed would be an independent, objective enquiry would show without doubt that they were not practising dangerously. The minutes of a Practice meeting at this time stated: 'Need to be very clear that we are very open to this enquiry... [we are] not shying away from an examination of our practice.'

Already very concerned about the misuse of the data in the Case Series, the midwives were anxious to know what evidence was being submitted to CEMACH to form the basis of its enquiry, how the enquiry would be carried out, and what question it was expected to answer. Pauline contacted Katie Yiannouzis on 11 February 2009 to try and clarify these points. On 17 February it was documented in the Practice minutes that Katie and Leonie 'know nothing about putting a question to CEMACH'. As both women had been central to the decision to commission the review, and they were both involved in the process of collecting and collating data and liaising with CEMACH, this seemed surprising. However, without any consultation with the midwives, a selection of their cases was sent to CEMACH.

Eventually, at a meeting on 3 March, the midwives were given some indication about what was being reviewed:

> 'CEMACH will scrutinise 33 cases, 11 from each of the following groups.
>
> Albany cases with poor outcome
>
> Albany control cases – the case immediately prior to the case with poor outcome
>
> Other cases where the baby developed HIE [there was no explanation of this last point]'

Over a period of eight months the midwives were given five different descriptions of the cases sent for review. In an email on 5 June Katie Yiannouzis stated that the 'Albany cases that went to CEMACH' were as follows:

> 12 cases – Albany cases with poor outcome (including the postnatal case)
>
> 11 cases – Albany control cases

There was no mention in this list of any other controls, either from the hospital or from other midwifery groups.

In the contract between King's and what had now become CMACE, which was sent to the midwives in September, it was stated that:

> 'KCH will provide 33 cases to be discussed in a confidential enquiry. There will be three comparison groups: 11 HIE cases from the Albany Practice; 11 HIE cases from KCH hospital-based care; and 11 controls (babies without HIE) from KCH hospital-based care. The controls will be matched to the Albany HIE cases by day of delivery.'

In a meeting in October the midwives told Katie Yiannouzis that they were still confused about which cases had been sent and asked whether the control cases were from the Albany or from King's. Katie replied that they included:

> Poor outcome from KCH
> Poor outcome from Albany
> Case before poor outcome from Albany

And finally, in a letter sent to the midwives in November from the Legal Services department at King's, just prior to the review being completed, it was stated that:

> 'CMACE carried out a review of 11 Albany cases with poor outcome, 11 Albany cases in which the outcome was "normal", and 11 cases from other King's group practices where the baby was admitted to the neonatal unit.'

In the event none of these five different descriptions was what actually happened. It is worth quoting here from the report itself, so that the disparity can clearly be seen.

> 'A series of 33 case records was provided to CMACE by the Trust, including:
> 11 cases relating to women who were cared for by the Albany Group Practice (AMP) whose babies had apparently suffered an intrapartum event leading to HIE and 1 case relating to a woman cared for by the AMP whose baby suffered hypoglycaemic brain injury (Group A)
> 10 cases relating to women cared for by the AMP whose babies did not have evidence of HIE (Group B)
> 11 cases from women cared for by other community based midwifery practices at King's (Group C) whose babies had unexpectedly required admission to the Neonatal Intensive Care Unit at King's College Hospital.'

It is difficult to comprehend why five different descriptions were given to the midwives, with not one of them being accurate. Why did this happen? What were communications like at King's and between King's and CEMACH and then CMACE? Was the contract between them drawn up at the start of the process or put together further down the line? And most importantly, how were the decisions made about which cases to include, and why did these appear to change so many times?

Meanwhile, having heard nothing following the meeting on 3 March, Pauline sent another letter to Sarah Dawson and Katie in May repeating the Practice's request for information about the review question. At a meeting on 1 June, Katie continued to deny any knowledge of this. However, she explained that CEMACH was looking into many different aspects of the midwives' care, such as whether or not King's guidelines were being followed, and whether or not the midwives were doing anything which might explain the poor outcomes. Sarah Dawson said that her understanding of the review remit was that it was to investigate whether or not the Practice as a whole was operating within King's guidelines, and whether or not King's' management processes were robust. All in all, it is perhaps an understatement to suggest that there was some confusion about what the review was intended to examine and accomplish.

To compound the confusion, on 5 June, Katie asked the midwives to go through their records and send a list of all Albany babies born in the 31-month period in question. This was in addition to King's 'trawling' through its database, and examining its Serious Untoward Incident reports and admissions to the Neonatal Unit. Katie explained that this was all being done in order to satisfy the midwives that the 'method of finding the cases is unbiased', although this had never been the real issue: it was how the cases had been used that was contested. The midwives continued to ask Katie for clarification about the enquiry. Eventually, in late June, they received an email from Rachel Thomas, the senior midwife overseeing the CEMACH review. She explained:

'We were approached by King's College Hospital to facilitate a peer review of a number of cases involving perinatal morbidity in a given timeframe.

'Contributors... have not been given any details about the Trust involved nor whether the cases involved are midwifery or obstetric led. In fact every effort has been made to maintain confidentiality to the extent that even most of the CEMACH staff do not know the Trust involved, as it is referred to as the "IP Project" only [a Panel member later remarked that it was obvious where the cases had come from]. Contributors are all external to the Trust and are a multidisciplinary mix of Obstetricians, Midwives, Independent Midwives and Neonatologists enabling a peer review of practice.'

The email went on to say:

'The panel members will be blinded to the outcome of the case to ensure they are not assessing the case with the benefit of hindsight. In addition the authors of the report will interview the Albany team and members of the maternity management team.'

It was a shock for the midwives to learn that they would be interviewed. This was the first time that they had heard about any interviews being part of the review. Pauline replied:

'Thank you for your email informing us that CEMACH would like to interview Albany midwives. We would like to be clear what the purpose of this is so late in the process, as we weren't expecting it. We would be glad if you could let us know why this has been suggested, what form it will take, who will be doing it and what questions the midwives will be facing so that they can prepare.'

Rachel replied, stating that 'details of the questions to be asked will not be available prior to the interviews'.

In the event, in July 2009 all the midwives were questioned individually about their practice by two members of the CMACE team. Each one of them found their interview traumatic, and Becky remembers being brought to tears by the experience.

The midwives had been told in January to expect the report within three to six months, but in the end it wasn't delivered to them until 30 November 2009. They had no idea what to expect from it, but assumed that it would have been rigorously carried out. However, alarm bells started ringing when they noticed that although it was described as 'A confidential enquiry into a series of term babies born in an unexpectedly poor condition', one of the Albany babies included in the review did not fit this category. He had been born in excellent condition, but became unwell two days later on the postnatal ward suffering from hypoglycaemia (low blood sugar). The Albany midwives were neither present nor responsible for this baby at the time of his collapse. Their request for him to be removed from the Case Series list had been agreed by Katie at a meeting in January, so the midwives were puzzled and dismayed to see this case included in the report. Why had CMACE included it? This did not bode well for the reliability or credibility of the report.

The process of the enquiry was described in the report as follows:

> 'The case records of all 33 women were anonymised then analysed by multidisciplinary enquiry panels of senior professionals including midwives from many specialties (including Supervisors of Midwives, Labour Ward Co-ordinators, Consultant Midwives, Independent Midwives, Midwifery Lecturers), Consultant Obstetricians, Consultant Neonatologists and Healthcare Managers drawn from across the UK. CMACE staff were present at all panel enquiries to ensure a consistent enquiry process and robust data collection. For each case, a semi-structured pro forma was completed which had previously been developed by CMACE and agreed with the Trust. This documented the consensus views of the panellists about the standards of care provided to women in the antenatal and intrapartum periods by both midwifery and medical staff. Panel assessors were blinded to the type of midwifery practice, name of the organisation and to the outcomes

of the babies in each case, whilst expressing their observations. The clinical condition of each baby was, however, revealed at the end of each case discussion so that the panellists could then state whether they thought that substandard care had contributed to the poor outcomes observed.'

The panels of six experts spent whole or half days reviewing cases using the tick box *pro forma* which had additional space for 'free text comments'. The panels allowed about an hour for each case, and although each review session might have had a different panel of experts, a non-participatory chairperson listened to proceedings and wrote a report using the day's paperwork.

Unsurprisingly, given the data they were working with, the report was unable to show any clear causal links between the Albany midwives' practice and the alleged poor clinical outcomes that had been the reason for the commissioning of the review. Instead the lengthy report contained a great number of observations, claims and commentary, including an eight-page section with 'a number of potentially useful observations'. The issues highlighted included:

The Albany way of working. The report stated that: 'this model of caseload working style compares unfavourably to other models of midwifery care, including other systems of caseload working, with respect to the volume and intensity of work that each midwife is exposed to'. It claimed that this caused physical and mental fatigue, which impacted on clinical judgement and that while it might be 'commendable [...], it may also generate more risk than it solves'.

The midwife-client relationship and women's choice. The report criticised the midwives' counselling of women, which 'appeared extreme in its non-directional manner' when the report stated that this should be more directive. At the same time it criticised them for appearing to influence women's decisions.

Place of birth. The report suggested that the midwives were supporting some women to have home births when it stated that they should have been strongly advised to give birth in hospital. It also criticised some hospital staff for being hostile towards the idea of home birth and not providing adequate support for the midwives.

Teamwork. The report suggested that the relationship between the Albany midwives and the hospital staff was antagonistic at times and not conducive to cohesive interdisciplinary team working.

Underlying the issues included in the report was the claim that the Albany midwives were not working within their Trust policies and guidelines, that they overlooked risk factors and possible complications during pregnancy and labour, that they required training to improve their level of competency, that they were working 'in isolation', and that their style of note-keeping was unsatisfactory and 'unusually graphic' because it included non-clinical observations, meaningful to the women but apparently unnecessary for clinicians.

The report ended with a detailed series of 'key recommendations' to improve both the Albany and King's working practices, and to improve communications between Albany midwives and staff at King's. These included:

- Reducing the midwives' workload, changing the midwives' 'working practices', and discontinuing the practice of accompanying women to consultations with other professionals.
- Introducing a 'homebirth risk assessment tool to determine whether it is safe for a woman to give birth at home'.
- Addressing system and attitudinal problems within the Trust such as the negative attitudes of some Trust staff towards the Albany midwives, community midwives and home birth.

Finally, it claimed that: 'addressing the key issues… would reduce the level of serious neonatal morbidity presently being encountered at King's College Hospital.'

The Albany midwives produced a response to the London

Project, explaining how the report had failed to understand their way of working, the concept of choice, and the role of the midwife. They explained that the report misrepresented their model of care: a model that had been well designed and researched, and found to work exceptionally well and to produce excellent health and satisfaction outcomes. They commented that 'no midwife ever worked for very long periods without support or relief'. Midwives were also able to manage their own workloads and had designated time off. They went on to note that 'this is in stark contrast with other group practices at KCH'.

The reviewers also appeared to misunderstand the concept of informed decision-making. During their interviews, each midwife was required to role play providing information to a woman about a specific urine test in pregnancy. Based on the interpretation of this role play the report had concluded that the midwives were too 'non-directional'. In relation to home birth, the report stated that: 'occasions will arise when definite, unequivocal and direct advice against homebirth is essential'. The midwives pointed out that this would have contravened the Code of Practice set out by their regulatory body, the Nursing and Midwifery Council, as well as the Royal College of Midwives' document 'Greater choice and control'. Both stated that the midwife should provide information so that women could make their own decisions. While Trust guidelines provide a framework for discussion, these do not override women's decisions, and midwives are required to support women whatever decisions they make. To do otherwise would be coercion.

The midwives were puzzled about the focus on home birth in the report. In only two of the Albany cases in which unexpectedly poor outcomes occurred was the baby born at home, although four were documented. This again served to undermine the midwives' confidence in the report's accuracy and reliability.

On the issue of teamwork, the report suggested that the Albany midwives worked in isolation and that there was almost no contact between the midwives and the hospital. The midwives explained that, on the contrary:

> *'The AMP had a good working relationship with Leonie Penna (link obstetrician), and referred women to other specialists when appropriate. The midwives cared for women on the Labour Ward alongside their hospital midwife colleagues, often supporting them if they were short-staffed. The AMP attended meetings with the midwifery managers, and the midwives were members of other hospital groups.'*

In response to the alleged lack of competency, the Albany midwives noted that many of the babies were under the care of medical staff at King's, and that of the seven competencies raised, only one was relevant to the outcomes of the babies. The midwives also commented that Albany babies had a consistently lower mortality rate than those in the surrounding area and that their outcomes were outstanding in an area of high disadvantage.

Finally, contradicting the view that the Albany midwives' case notes were inadequate because they contained descriptive as well as clinical detail, the results of a case note audit at King's carried out during the investigation period found that Albany midwives met the standard 'fully and consistently', and that there were examples of 'exemplary documentation'. In other parts of King's maternity services, it was found that 'there is room for considerable improvement in documentation standards'.

In their response, the Albany midwives suggested that the reviewer's observations were largely based on lack of knowledge about their practice and outcomes, and on subjective opinion rather than any recognised evidence.

Perhaps due to the esteem in which the Albany Practice was held, and the overwhelming support for the AMP model of care, several responses criticising the CMACE Report were written. King's initially tried to keep the report confidential. However, in the third week of December, Denis Walsh, Associate Professor of Midwifery at Nottingham University, wrote in an email to a senior midwife at King's: 'I have been sent the CMACE Report by a journalist. I know it is confidential but I am writing a critique of it...'

By January 2010 others had obtained copies of the report via Freedom of Information* requests, and in March critiques were produced by both the NCT and AIMS. The main criticisms included that the report lacked context to support the claims it made, that the methodology and processes used were flawed in various ways, that there was no acknowledgement of the problematic nature of the term HIE and how it was defined and used, and that parts of the report relied too heavily on subjective opinion.

The CEMACH/CMACE panellists were provided with very little context to assist them in reaching their conclusions about the Albany Midwifery Practice, and making the observations that they did. As the critiques explained, there was no reference made to the Albany Practice's previous excellent evaluations, or to its very low mortality rates in comparison to those of other King's babies. AIMS pointed out:

> 'The introduction of the CMACE Report refers to the excellent reputation of King's Maternity Unit, but fails to balance this by referring to previous evaluations of the Albany Midwifery Practice that demonstrated excellent outcomes and satisfaction (Sandall et al 2001, Rosser 2003). Nor does it mention a report by Jill Demilew (Consultant Midwife at King's), showing the many benefits to women and babies provided by the community midwifery practices including the Albany Midwifery Practice (Demilew 2007). This lack of balance gives an unfortunate impression of bias at the beginning of the CMACE Report. Is it possible that the CMACE team was not made aware of these three reports?'

Denis Walsh made a similar observation, pointing out that the AMP was cited in an extract from the King's Fund Report on Maternity Care Safety entitled *Safe Births* (2008) which stated that

---

* The Freedom of Information Act (2000) gave members of the public the right to access information held by public authorities, including government departments, local authorities, the NHS, state schools and police forces.

'it is possible to achieve high rates of productivity and excellent outcomes with the AMP's innovative model of care'. It is ironic that this was published in the same year that the safety of the Albany Practice was being called into question by King's. As Denis commented: 'The reviewers seem completely blind to the previous success of this model and its citation in many journal papers and other reports'.

Both AIMS and the NCT commented on the apparent bias embedded in the enquiry from the outset. The AIMS critique said: 'King's set the time frame, and King's selected the cases. The basis on which they were chosen is not given anywhere.' More worryingly, CMACE appeared to accept King's' assertion that Albany babies had an increased incidence of HIE, stating in the report that:

> 'The hospital had identified that over a 31 month period the number of admissions of term infants with serious morbidities including hypoxic-ischaemic encephalopathy (HIE) was comparatively 10 fold greater amongst women under the care of the Albany Group Practice than women cared for by other King's midwifery group practices or by hospital midwives.'

The report contained no evidence or explanation for this statement. As no adequate comparison was ever made between Albany babies and babies born to women receiving care from the hospital or other midwifery practices at King's, this couldn't have been proved either way. As the AIMS critique pointed out, it 'excluded the possibility that the adverse outcomes identified could have been misdiagnosed, or have occurred by chance'. It also excluded the possibility that in the context of overall outcomes a different interpretation might have emerged.

Those criticising the report noted another potential element of bias. A statement in the report claimed that the reviewers were not told the outcomes of the cases that they were examining in order to avoid 'hindsight bias', but several commentators noticed that this was not the case. They pointed out that although the case records were reviewed anonymously by the panels, each of the baby's clinical conditions was revealed before the reviewers judged whether or not the care was substandard. As Denis Walsh explained:

> 'Though reviewers were blinded to outcome when reviewing the case, they were not blinded up to the point of their recommendation of whether substandard care contributed to outcome. After reviewing care, they were then told the outcome before submitting a recommendation. This exposed them to hindsight bias, well known in the literature to affect retrospective review (Zain et al 1998). The true test of judgement is to make a recommendation on the care that is reviewed whilst not knowing the outcome.'

In other words, the CMACE process introduced bias through the 'benefit of hindsight', which it had previously stated it wanted to avoid.

The critiques questioned whether the methodology used was appropriate for such a small number of cases. In the words of the report, the purpose of confidential enquiry methodology was: 'to determine whether and to what extent there is a pattern of recurrent avoidable factors associated with adverse outcomes in a care system'. But as AIMS commented, this is 'designed to look for trends in large groups of cases in order to help to identify practice changes to improve outcomes'. There was no explanation about why CMACE used this methodology to compare the outcomes of a small number of cases, or why it didn't use a more appropriate methodology such as root cause analysis, which is designed to examine individual cases in depth.

It transpired later that CMACE had planned to statistically analyse the data sent by King's. A midwife who was a member of the CMACE Panels expressed her concerns about this in a later interview. She reported how another Panel member had said, 'we need figures to give to the Trust... King's need stats, that's what they want, figures, because there's going to be an outcome to this.' She felt incredulous that 'they were using statistics, you know, percentages and p-values. And I remember just going hot and cold, thinking I've got to say something.' In the end she did, and it was thanks to her that there were no statistics in the final report, which said:

> 'After careful consideration, tests of statistical significance were not applied to the data since the methodological features of the enquiry precluded such an approach... the reader must appreciate that the study methodology employed does not lend itself to meaningful statistical analysis.'

It is worrying, nevertheless, that a statistical analysis of descriptive data was ever considered.

The notion of a cluster was raised yet again. No definition of this was provided in the report, but as we have seen, clusters are difficult to identify and even if they are they are unlikely to be significant. As AIMS pointed out 'it is unclear whether 12 babies over a particular 31 months would constitute a "cluster".'

There had been criticisms of the unusual time frame used in the Case Series and the internal audit, and the same concerns were expressed in critiques of the CMACE Report. However, the report itself made no comment on this.

The use of the term 'HIE' was also questioned, and commentators asked why the report had not discussed its complexities, why it had not defined it, and why it had accepted the assumption that it was the result of poor care. On this last point, Denis Walsh made the important observation that:

> 'HIE has an incidence of about 2.5 per 1,000 in term infants. In other words, in a hospital of 6,000 births, 12–14 cases per year. Only about 15% of these are related to intrapartum events as the vast majority are known to be linked to antenatal causation. Thus

out of 12–14 cases in a 6,000 birth hospital, about 2 cases will be related to intrapartum events. That is why any review would not expect to conclude that of the 11 cases of HIE from Albany, most were down to intrapartum events. A 'quick and dirty' review like this one (and CMACE admit the limitations of this review at the beginning of the document) is not detailed and thorough enough to make these judgements and is almost certainly misleading in its conclusions on this basis alone.'

In addition, the CMACE panellists not only accepted King's' diagnosis of HIE in Albany babies, but they also provided no definition or grading of it. Nor did they make any comment about King's' apparent failure to provide two-year follow-up data for the babies diagnosed with HIE. This had been a requirement since 2006, when the National Neonatal Audit was set up by the Royal College of Paediatrics and Child Health to monitor and improve the care of babies admitted to Special Care Baby Units across the country.

The Albany midwives' and others' view, that the report was largely based on bias and opinion, was supported by comments made in a later interview with one of the CMACE Panel members. She said 'I assumed that the process they were using was a tried and tested, evaluated, hard and fast [process]' and believed that 'they must know what they're doing'. She was alarmed by the lack of consistency of the panels as panellists came and went: 'some people just came for the afternoon'. Obstetricians and neonatologists would 'run in the door' probably without having looked at the cases. She expressed concern about the ad hoc nature of the panel makeup and the resulting lack of robustness of the process. She found that the 'consensus views of the panellists' were very opinion-based, and that the process 'just didn't feel rigorous really... I sort of felt it became more based on people's opinion. I was quite shocked by how unevidence based it was.'

This panel member also described specific incidents that she felt compromised the findings of the report. On more than one occasion the midwifery risk manager from King's who had compiled the data on the Albany babies joined the enquiry panels, supposedly as a 'gagged' observer. The panellist was shocked when the manager 'piped up a couple of times. And at that point, I said to the person who was running it "That can't happen again, seriously, that's affecting the impartiality of the whole process..."'.

Putting aside its innumerable shortcomings, King's had repeatedly told the midwives that any decisions about the future of their practice would be based on the findings and recommendations of the CMACE Report. Nowhere in the report was it suggested that the Albany Midwifery Practice should be closed. As Denis Walsh remarked:

> 'the review does not recommend the termination of the contract, but a series of ameliorative measures to improve the working relationships, clinical governance and training at the group's interface with the hospital.'

In April 2010 the chair of AIMS, Beverley Beech, wrote to the chair of CMACE, Professor James Walker, questioning the quality of the report and the subsequent closure of the Albany Midwifery Practice. He replied:

> 'A number of recommendations were made based primarily on the findings of the panels. The actions subsequently taken by the Trust, which did not include adoption of our recommendations, are a matter for them to explain' [authors' emphasis]

All the recommendations in this expensive and time-consuming report were ignored in the end. In spite of the claim that any decision about the future of the Albany Midwifery Practice would be based on the findings of the CMACE Report, a decision was quickly made by King's to close the Practice down.

Mavis Kirkham
Midwifery Professor Emerita, Sheffield Hallam University

The closure of the Albany Practice is a tragedy which says a great deal about the state of the NHS and particularly the management of NHS maternity services.

The Albany demonstrated what can be done for families and for midwives. Good practice and excellent clinical outcomes were achieved through relationships, not by the proliferation of rules. They followed the traditional midwifery model where midwives are with women and committed to their care, rather than prioritising the detailed requirements of their employing organisation.

The Albany midwives facilitated antenatal groups which enabled women to build the friendships which would sustain them later as mothers. The groups and the one-to-one antenatal education helped women to develop confidence in their ability to birth their babies and worked to dispel the fear which is now so common around birth. The time the Albany midwives spent with their mothers antenatally meant that these mothers were well prepared for labour, birth and motherhood.

The Albany mothers felt well supported, had confidence in themselves and supported each other. This is rare in our modern NHS. Maternity services have been starved and diminished to the point where monitoring, rather than care, is prioritised to protect the organisation. Technology is therefore seen as essential, fear is widespread, and staffing reduced. Thus relationships are discounted. In this climate, midwifery management cannot model the care and support skills for midwives which they in turn can use to make such a difference for mothers. Indeed midwifery managers have to closely control their workforce to meet the requirements of higher management and to plug gaps in the depleted service. Excellent practice can be seen as a threat rather than an example of what can be achieved. Innovation is not encouraged and tall poppies are scythed.

It is ironic that the Albany Practice was probably the most researched and evaluated midwifery practice in the world. Its clinical outcomes were beyond dispute. The love the mothers felt for it was shown in the demonstrations against the closure. It is often cited as a birth model that worked and as an example of excellence in UK midwifery practice. Its closure suggests that the current UK birth model is not working. Its spirit lives on in the mothers and midwives to whom it showed what is possible. My daughter is one of the many student midwives to whom the Albany was an inspiration.

13

Salama's story: 'the straw that broke the camel's back'

Throughout 2009, while CMACE was slowly and laboriously putting together its report, and while all the other various measures were in place, the midwives continued their day-to-day work. Whatever was going on behind the scenes, the women of Peckham continued to be looked after. Bookings, antenatal visits, births and postnatal care continued as normal despite the cloud of suspicion hanging over the midwives.

In April Becky met and booked Salama (not her real name), who was expecting her third baby. Becky explained that she and one other midwife, Fran, would be looking after Salama throughout her pregnancy, birth and postnatal period, offering total continuity of carer. Salama had given birth at home in Sierra Leone to her first baby 'with her mum and midwife helping', and had had her second baby in King's Hospital with no problems. In view of this Becky discussed with her the option of choosing a home birth this time, and she said she would like that if all went well.

The booking visit at Salama's home was a joyful occasion. Her friend Eshe (not her real name) was with her, and her husband Salim (not his real name) and their young daughter were also in the flat. Becky took a photo of Salama lying with her head on Eshe's lap as she waited for Becky to check her, both of them smiling broadly at the camera. Everyone was excited and happy as they looked forward to this much-wanted new baby. A plan of care was discussed, including antenatal visits with both Becky and Fran, a referral to an obstetrician if any problems arose, and then hopefully both midwives being with Salama for her birth. As with almost all women offered this model of midwifery care, Salama was very happy to know that she would have midwives that she knew looking after her. A scan had already been arranged for the following month, and Becky made another antenatal appointment with Salama before she said goodbye.

Midwives are only too aware that nothing is predictable in their profession, and what was about to unfold was something that no one would have imagined. As we have seen, King's' hypothesis about the safety of the Albany Practice had already been formed and Salama's story was to 'fit' that hypothesis, and become pivotal in the story of the AMP.

Salama had a straightforward pregnancy. She remained well and her baby grew beautifully. Her 'due date' of 14 September came and went, but Salama remained relaxed and very keen to have her planned home birth. A scan at 41 weeks and 4 days showed that everything appeared normal. Salama decided that she would like to have her labour induced at 42 weeks if she hadn't given birth by then, so this was arranged with the hospital.

The day before Salama's planned induction Becky rang her to arrange a home visit to check all was well. Salama didn't want a visit but did say that she wanted to go into labour that night as she really didn't want to go to hospital. Becky arranged to ring Salama the following morning with a time to meet her at King's for the induction. Salama repeated that she really wanted to have her baby at home.

Salama went into spontaneous labour later that night. After receiving her call, Becky and Laura (a student midwife from Australia on placement with the Practice) arrived at the flat at 3.45am, and Salama's baby girl was born normally at 5.51am. There were no problems in the labour, and no indications at all of the tragedy that was about to happen. Salama's baby, born in good condition and cuddled by Salama as she rang her mother in Sierra Leone, collapsed suddenly at 25 minutes old. Resuscitation was started immediately, and within eight minutes an ambulance had arrived to transfer the baby to hospital. By the time the baby was admitted to the neonatal intensive care unit her condition was described as 'very poor', the doctors were considering discontinuing her life support, and the consultant on call had been asked to come in from home before any decisions were taken.

Of course, tragedies can and do happen in birth, and it is often impossible to foresee such events. There were three midwives and a student in the flat that night: the fallout from the events at Salama's birth was to touch all of them in different ways, but its impact on the Albany Practice itself was profound. Given the situation that the AMP was in at the time, Becky's reaction as the baby collapsed is perhaps not surprising. At the same time as immediately going into emergency response mode and initiating resuscitation, she remembers experiencing a simultaneous awareness of the implications that this awful situation would have for the Practice. It really did feel like the proverbial straw that was very likely to break the camel's back.

In the hospital Salama and Salim were in shock, and distraught about what was happening to their newborn daughter. Although the doctors were painting a very bleak picture indeed, and explaining that she was in a very serious condition and unlikely to survive without severe brain damage, Salama and Salim were not yet ready to take the decision to turn off her life support. Understandably they wanted their baby to have every chance. It was therefore arranged for the baby to be transferred to another hospital for a therapy known as 'controlled cooling', in which the baby's body (and brain) is cooled in the hope of slowing down the processes that cause brain damage. However, after a few days it was obvious that the baby was showing no signs of improvement, and Salama and Salim understood that she was not going to recover. With their agreement her intensive care support was discontinued, and she died in Salama's arms shortly afterwards.

Meanwhile the response from King's was immediate and devastating. The morning after Salama's birth a message was received at the Practice to say that Katie and Leonie would be visiting for an emergency meeting. When they arrived the tone was judgemental and accusatory, with no sympathy at all expressed for the midwives who had had such a traumatic time the day before. Everyone knew that what had happened was extremely unusual and difficult to explain. But from Katie and Leonie there was an immediate assumption of blame, and almost unbelievably they challenged the midwives' version of events. Leonie even questioned whether Salama really had held her baby, suggesting that the baby must have been in such poor condition at birth that this would have been impossible. But Becky had taken a photo of Salama on the phone to her mother, with her baby in her arms. It seemed that what had happened fitted so well with the narrative at the time, that even clear provable facts were being disputed and replaced with 'alternative facts'. Katie and Leonie interpreted events in a way that confirmed their existing beliefs about the safety of the Practice, a perfect example of 'confirmation bias'.

Katie and Leonie brought a letter to the meeting from Sarah Dawson, the Divisional Manager for Women's and Children's Services, stating that, following the unexpected adverse outcome at Salama's birth, 'we have serious concerns regarding the safety of the home birth service provided by Albany'. This was a new slant, although not entirely unexpected. Although the original Case Series list had indeed commented on place of birth, this had been removed in the second and third versions. And yet, as discussed earlier, there did seem to be a genuine fear among King's obstetricians that home birth was inherently dangerous. A later comment by one of them was to highlight this. In a conversation with a woman booked with another group practice, who was considering having a home birth, she said that although the woman didn't have any specific contraindication to home birth, 'nobody is suitable for it and nobody should be considering it'.

The 'serious concerns' in Sarah Dawson's letter had led to what felt like a catastrophic knee-jerk reaction from the Trust to Salama's birth. The letter went on to say:

'The Trust has decided that we have no option but to suspend the Albany home birth service pending the outcome of the CEMACH enquiry and the investigation into this case.

With immediate effect, all women booked under Albany will need to attend hospital for labour assessments and deliveries. Women wishing to have a home birth from now until mid-November will still be accommodated by King's but will need to transfer to another group practice for their care... The provision of antenatal and postnatal care is unaffected by the suspension of the home birth service.'

So there it was. A decision had been taken without any evidence of malpractice and before any enquiry, and without even hearing the midwives' story: it was to be implemented 'with immediate effect'. The midwives protested but were powerless. As soon as Katie and Leonie had left and the midwives had picked themselves up, they began to plan how to inform all the women booked with them of the decision, and how to deal with the inevitable consequences. Women were now going to have to choose between birthing with midwives they knew and trusted, but not in a place of their choosing, or continuing to plan to give birth at home with midwives they didn't know and had never met. One woman wrote in a post on a local social media forum: 'I'm in a dilemma. Want a homebirth but want the midwife from Albany who I've seen for the last 8 months'.

It was no surprise that all the women who had either reached their due date or were approaching it decided to stay with their Albany midwives, stating that having a known midwife with them in labour was more important to them than their place of birth. Some of these women became very angry about the situation, and eventually added their voices to the Albany mums' campaign (see Chapter 16).

Salama's baby had been born on a Monday morning. On Friday evening, with no prior warning, Becky was summoned to an emergency meeting via a call on her pager. Not surprisingly she felt very apprehensive, and asked Zoe to attend with her for support. She also contacted Cathy Walton, who had already left the hospital at the end of her working day. Cathy was on her way to her home outside London, but willingly turned round and made her way back to be at the meeting. As Becky left her house she bumped into her friend who was working for the Audit Commission, on her way home from work. She saw Becky's obvious distress and insisted on accompanying her to the hospital, where Katie Yiannouzis and Sarah Dawson were waiting.

Becky had been right to be concerned, as the meeting had been called in order to suspend her from duty. Becky and Zoe asked to record the meeting and were surprised when Katie and Sarah agreed. Katie appeared nervous and hesitant, and took a while to get to the point. She accused Becky of being 'in an emotional state that may make you possibly not make the right decisions', and suggested that she could 'take some leave'. When Becky didn't answer immediately Katie went on:

> 'if you're not prepared to take any leave then I've asked you to come here to tell you that I don't want you to look after any more King's women until we... resolve this. So I'm in effect suspending you from duty... okay? [...] And I think perhaps I need to explain that suspension is a neutral act, it's a neutral act [...] and it's for your protection as much as for King's while the investigations are completed [...] just to lift you out of the situation.'

For Becky this action definitely didn't feel like a 'neutral act'. She felt the implication of blame just as she had felt it three days earlier, after the meeting with Katie and Leonie at the Practice. An employment law solicitor has said that 'Suspension from duty [...] inevitably casts a shadow over the employee's competence. Of course this does not mean that it cannot be done, but it is not a neutral act.'*

---

* www.footanstey.com/article/suspension-a-neutral-act

Talking about what happened to the Albany Midwifery Practice and more generally about the way practitioners are treated when adverse incidents occur, Jane Sandall commented: 'It's awful, whether it's a midwife or a doctor, it's just awful. You know the level of support is not there. Then comes the scapegoating...'. She suggested that while there is some support in place for doctors:

> 'there is nothing for nurses and midwives. And the response is so often [...] to suspend people... by suspending someone, and sending them off duty, even when you don't know – how could you know what's happened at that point, because it happens immediately – is a disaster for that person. They're isolated, it's punitive, there's blaming. It's absolutely tragic...'

Becky was indeed being sent off duty, without having had the opportunity to explain her side of the story. The meeting continued with questions from Zoe about why Becky was being singled out for suspension when she hadn't been the only midwife at Salama's birth, and what support the Trust would be offering to the Practice while Becky wasn't allowed to work. Katie mumbled that there would be managers on call, and ended the meeting saying she was going on holiday for two weeks the following morning.

That same day King's started a supervisory investigation into Becky's practice. It was a detailed and protracted process, very painful at times, ending in the recommendation that Becky undergo a period of supervised practice in another Trust (see Chapter 20).

Following any serious adverse outcome in maternity care, a root cause analysis risk management investigation should be carried out by the relevant Trust. This process was started by King's following Salama's birth. The report arising from this investigation was submitted to the Maternity Risk Management Group on Christmas Eve 2009. It contained seven 'recommendations for action and learning'. Although this was not communicated to Becky at the time, the final recommendation was that she should be referred by the Head of Midwifery Katie Yiannouzis to the Nursing and Midwifery Council, the midwives' regulatory body.

Following Salama's birth, Becky was told by King's not to have any further contact with the family. In a meeting with one of the neonatal consultants to discuss what had happened, Salama and her husband were informed that the baby 'had had a period of about 2 hours before she was born in which she had had a lack of oxygen, and that because of this she had brain damage'. Although there was no evidence for this opinion, it led the parents to believe that the midwives had been at fault. With this in mind, they employed a lawyer and a lengthy formal complaint about their midwifery care was submitted to the Trust the following April.

In early spring 2011, almost a year and a half after Salama's birth, an inquest was finally held into the death of her baby. It had been planned for May 2010 but had been cancelled, due to 'the Coroner being involved in a number of lengthy inquests'. However, although the inquest itself was yet another painful process to go through, for Becky the final outcome was positive. She was of course called to give evidence, and the coroner stated that she found Becky to be 'an honest and credible witness'.

A consultant obstetrician who was appointed as an expert witness for the parents suggested that asphyxia can occur in the last few weeks of pregnancy as well as during labour. Following the post mortem the baby's brain had been sent for further expert analysis, the findings of which supported this view. The post mortem investigation had revealed signs of chronic hypoxia, and the pathologist at the inquest had attempted to date this. She said that the calcification seen in the baby's brain was likely to have been present for 'in the region of seven days', which would suggest that hypoxia had commenced approximately two days before the birth. Clearly this meant that in the pathologist's opinion the baby's death could not have been predicted, and was not caused by any failure of care on the part of the midwives. In her summing up the coroner said:

> 'I am going to record a conclusion that [the baby's] death was due
> to the effects of chronic hypoxia commencing about two days prior
> to delivery...'

By this time, and based primarily on this case, Becky was undergoing
the maximum length of supervised practice – 450 hours – at a
hospital in north London, far from her home. She had been given
time off to attend the inquest, and the following day she wrote to
thank the Head of Midwifery for agreeing to this.

> 'The inquest was a gruelling couple of days, but it's over and with
> a good result. The coroner gave a short narrative verdict, finding
> no evidence of neglect. It was found that the baby had had an
> antenatal hypoxic insult, which we could not have diagnosed [...]
> As you can imagine I'm relieved it's over and very relieved at the
> findings.'

However, even with the inquest findings, there was no suggestion
of calling a halt to Becky's supervised practice.

Katie Yiannouzis had referred Becky to the NMC over a year
earlier, based on this very case. She was present at the inquest,
sitting just behind Becky. She refused to make eye contact and
made no comment after the verdict was read out.

Salama was also present, and this was the first time she and
Becky had met since her baby's birth. In the court they were unable
to talk, but outside, as Salama was being driven away, she wound
down her window and called out to Becky: 'I'm sorry. I never
wanted it to be like this'.

14
Closure

'It really is sad that something that could have had such a positive influence on the profession was snuffed out in such a political and uninformed fashion.' Albany dad

Not surprisingly, after the home birth service was terminated at the end of September 2009, and Becky suspended in October, the Practice experienced even more turmoil and confusion. The midwives felt yet again that they were living and working in a parallel universe. Although they continued to receive support from many quarters, there was an increasing feeling of impending doom, with continued long delays to the publication of the CMACE Report, and to the conclusion of the internal audit.

Practical issues took up much of the midwives' time: how to run the Practice with one midwife unable to work, how to keep women and their families informed and up to date with what the Practice could offer them, and how to handle the continuing requests for visits from midwives and students wanting to learn about the Albany model of care.

By 13 October, the Trust had still not provided any written information for the women being looked after by the Albany Practice. The midwives felt strongly that, having closed the home birth service with no warning, it was the responsibility of King's to inform the women. So, on behalf of the midwives, Zoe and Mary wrote to Sarah Dawson expressing their concern that women would find out about the home birth suspension from other women or at the antenatal and postnatal groups, and how unsatisfactory this was.

Concern about how to do the day-to-day work of the Practice was at the forefront of the midwives' minds. The Albany model was being severely compromised. In an emotional meeting with

Katie Yiannouzis on 22 October the midwives repeatedly asked for guidance. They explained that they were unable to recruit 'due to the current situation', and were worried about not fulfilling their contract. Katie replied: 'We put you in this position; you are not in breach of contract... we can't expect you to fulfill your contract if you haven't got all the midwives.' When asked about continuing to do bookings, Katie replied that they should 'do what they can'. It seemed that the Head of Midwifery was finding it difficult to respond to any of the midwives' concerns, and was abdicating her responsibility for the safe running of the maternity services.

Meanwhile, feeling increasingly desperate about the problems with the original Case Series data, Becky was spending all her time agonising over what could possibly be done to improve the situation for the Practice. Following a support meeting at Becky's house (described in Chapter 18), Mavis Kirkham wrote to Professor Alison Macfarlane on 26 October, asking her if she would look at the statistics that had been used to question the safety of the midwives' practice. In her email to Alison she said:

> *'The statistics of this sound very dodgy, no one is disputing that their mortality figures are lower than those for King's and the locality. This feels like real witch-hunting and the Practice will be lost unless something can be done very soon.'*

Understanding the urgency of the situation, Alison replied immediately, and Becky and Pauline met with her at City University the following day. Having anonymised the Case Series, they took with them the three different versions and asked Alison for her opinion.

Alison immediately committed herself to working on the Case Series data, and in the middle of November she produced the comprehensive paper discussed in Chapter 9 titled 'Comments on case series from King's College Hospital'. It is worth repeating Alison's main finding, which was that from the data provided 'it is impossible to draw any inferences'. And very importantly, given that this Case Series was the evidence that was sent to CEMACH and was the basis upon which they unquestioningly conducted their investigation, Alison commented: 'The lack of definitions and inclusion criteria call into question these case series as a sampling frame for any investigations to be undertaken in greater depth.'

And yet of course that is exactly what had happened, and by the time that Alison wrote this the report was done and dusted and on its way to King's.

Later in November, still feeling a serious lack of support or direction from management, Pauline wrote to Katie:

> 'We are really concerned that we have been trying for some while now to organise a meeting to discuss how we as a Practice can continue... we want to urgently discuss the provision of care for women... We have women booked to the end of May as if we are a full service, i.e. six whole caseload equivalents. We are informing you of this situation as our contracts manager and Head of the Midwifery Service and would like an urgent response as to how the Trust plans to take this forward.'

In a dismissive reply, Katie thanked Pauline for reminding her of 'the concerns of the Albany midwives', saying she had realised that some of the midwives were in the hospital that afternoon and had organised a meeting with them and with Kate Brintworth. She said: 'I explained to them how recently established caseload groups [at King's] have worked in their early days when they did not have six midwives', and that she expected 'something similar' from the Albany: 'They need to... between them do all the antenatals and postnatals. We are not expecting them to cover labour care.'

During the months of October and November the midwives continued to nervously await the CMACE Report. The timeline for the publication of the report had changed many times over the course of the year. Having been told in early March that the report was 'expected by the end of June', it was now months later and the delay in its arrival was starting to make the midwives feel not only anxious, but also somewhat suspicious. They had been told, after all, that decisions about the future of the Albany Practice would be dependent on its findings. At the end of September Sarah Dawson had written to say that King's was not expecting to receive the 'outcome of the CMACE review' until 31 October. On 30 October Sarah Dawson wrote again, informing the Practice of a further delay:

> 'I was expecting it this weekend but they have told me it will be delayed until the 11th November. I will be in a position to report to Albany on the morning of the 16th November and Katie and I would like to meet with the Practice on the morning of the 17th November.'

Suspicion was growing in the Practice about the delay between King's receiving the report and the Albany having sight of it. The midwives and Pauline were starting to suspect that King's might be having some input into what they thought was an independent report, albeit in its final stages. Pauline replied:

> 'We have been informed that the King's management staff have been meeting with CMACE on the report before the report has been finalised. In the interests of transparency, can you provide promptly details of what discussions you have had to date.'

In reply to Pauline's email, Sarah Dawson said: 'We need to read and digest the report and subject it to our own governance processes', and continued:

> 'In relation to our conversations with CMACE, as you would expect the people we have commissioned to provide us with an independent report have briefed us periodically on progress. I do not think it is appropriate to share this with you until I see the full report as I do not know what will be included.'

Although the AMP had no details of any meetings, it was clear that there had been ongoing communication between King's and CMACE. In a confidential briefing from 'the Division' (presumably

Maternity) for King's Executive, written on 16 November and obtained via a Freedom of Information request, it was stated that 'verbal updates on the progress of the review have been discussed at the Trust's Governance Committee on the 23rd April, 23rd July and 22nd October.'

Time dragged on, with dates continually changing and everyone in the Practice becoming increasingly nervous and exasperated. Finally, on 23 November, an email was received from Tim Smart, the Chief Executive at King's:

> 'I am writing to inform you that the CMACE report will not be available for release as planned on Monday 23rd November as it needs to be reviewed and considered by the Trust Board before being shared. The Trust will send the report to the Albany Practice on Monday 30th November. I apologise for this further delay but as you can appreciate, delays until this point have been outside the Trust's control.'

That afternoon Pauline wrote to Sarah Dawson, saying 'You might imagine the distress and dismay this is causing us. I have tried to ring you to discuss how we continue in this situation for yet another week.' Becky also wrote to Francine Allen, the RCM representative, that same afternoon, saying 'We are shocked and appalled at yet another prolongation of our distress and insecurity'.

Finally, in the early evening of Monday 30 November, a hard copy of the CMACE Report (bizarrely titled 'The London Project') was delivered to the Albany Practice. Having had confirmation from Sarah Dawson that the report would finally be sent by courier that afternoon, the midwives were all gathered together in their meeting room in Peckham Pulse. This was the culmination of many weeks of waiting, and everyone was feeling apprehensive and emotional. The courier arrived, the large brown envelope was handed over, and the slightly hysterical midwives took photos even before they dared to open it. It would take some time for them to unscramble and make sense of its contents, but the main finding

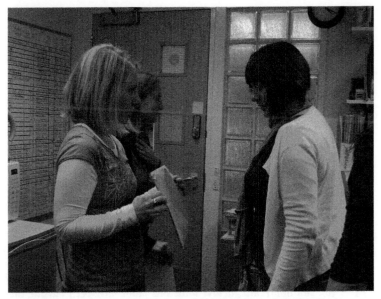

Midwives Nicky, Zoe and Fran with the long-awaited CMACE Report

that they were able to deduce from an initial reading that day was that there was no recommendation to close the Practice.

Meanwhile, the midwives had been thinking of other ways of holding the Trust to account. In early November they met with a barrister to look at whether there was any possible action that could be taken. Eleena listened carefully to the story, and then put together a 'letter before action', requiring the Trust to respond to questions about the contract, the ongoing investigation into the Practice, the suspension of the home birth service, Becky's suspension from duty, and the consequent reputational damage to the Albany Practice. The letter also queried the fact that the CMACE review 'is proceeding with missing data', saying: 'This is plainly unsatisfactory and suggests a dereliction of duty on the part of the Trust to its clients.' The legal department at King's responded swiftly but unhelpfully, failing to answer some of the questions. Given what would unfold a fortnight or so later, the following statement included in their reply was particularly interesting:

> '*It has never been the intention of the Trust to cause or contribute to reputational damage of the Albany or individual midwives… The actions it has taken to date have been with the primary objective of ensuring the safety of the women under the Albany's care* and to support the Albany to continue practising' [our emphasis].

Alongside all the difficulties, however, more positive things were happening. On 11 November the report on the Birth Talks was finally delivered to the Practice by Jill Demilew, one of the report authors. This report had been set in motion almost a year earlier as part of the special measures imposed on the Albany midwives, and was titled '*Report of Review of 36 week 'Birth Talk', an Observational Audit (December 2008 – August 2009)*'. The aim, as described by Katie, had been: 'To ensure that the 36 week birth talk is completed to expected standards for all women including low risk women'. Given the implied concern at the very start of the whole process that the midwives might be supporting women to make dangerous decisions, the outcome of this audit was seen by many to be a crucial piece of evidence. The two consultant midwives responsible for the report, Jill Demilew and Cathy Walton, had developed the following standard against which to assess their observations:

> '*[That] all women have the opportunity at 36 weeks to discuss their options and choices for labour and birth taking into account any identified risk factors linked with possible increased poorer outcomes and in the context of any relevant […] guidance. [And that] the documentation provides clear evidence of the information shared, decisions made and care planned.*'

An audit tool was developed based on these standards, and an assessment process, consisting of observations of 26 birth talks, was carried out over an eight-month period. The findings were emphatic and clear:

> 'The Trust can be assured that at the conclusion of this audit,
> the Albany midwives met the above standard and are providing
> a high standard of care. Exemplary practice was noted regarding
> information sharing and discussion of women's wishes and
> preferences. Risk factors were identified and consultation and/or
> referral with a consultant obstetrician always occurred.'

As part of their observational audit the authors had carried out
a 'snapshot audit' of maternity records of a comparative cohort
of women on one day in the postnatal ward at King's, using the
same audit tool, in order to 'give the context of the standards of
documentation around information sharing and planning for
birth in the wider maternity service.' Their findings were starkly
different from those above, showing that, for example, in 11% of
cases 'the risks and benefits of place of birth were very poorly
documented', and in 7% of cases 'documentation of monitoring
fetal wellbeing in labour was particularly poorly documented'. And
for more than two-thirds of women, their wishes and preferences
for labour were not documented at all. The authors concluded:
'The findings from the Snapshot audit suggest that there is room
for considerable improvement in documentation standards in other
parts of the maternity service.'

Sadly, the results of this eagerly awaited Birth Talk audit arrived
too late, if indeed they were ever going to influence the outcome.
By mid-November a decision about the future of the Albany
Practice had probably already been made. Whether or not this was
the case, letters and emails in support of the Albany continued to
arrive at King's. Dr Mark Ashworth, a Peckham GP and Medical
Director, who in May 2008 had taken over responsibility for one of
the GP practices referring pregnant women to the Albany Practice,
wrote to Tim Smart on 25 November, saying that he had been
'tremendously impressed by the Albany Midwife team'. In a long
and persuasive letter, he detailed his reasons for being moved to
write in support:

'In a community with a high perinatal and infant mortality, the Albany Midwives provide, in my opinion, a vital service. Their strong points are their access (they assertively seek out all the many non-attenders for antenatal care) and their professionalism (I have learnt a lot from my contact with the team and all my patients report the very highest standards). Their home delivery service has always been of the highest standard and I have personally seen many patients who cannot praise the team highly enough for their dedication and professional care.'

Having highlighted what he called the 'strong points' of the Practice, Dr Ashworth made the following stark observation: 'What I do know is that without their assertive outreach and home delivery service, many of the women who I see who live on the margins of society would simply have no care at all.'

The letter continued with a plea to Tim Smart, asking him to 'take some note of the viewpoint of our general practice which tries to engage with the very same community, and also of the local community itself which holds the Albany Midwives in great respect.' This was a very powerful endorsement which was shamefully ignored by the decision-makers at King's.

In November 2009, the newly formed campaign group known as the Albany Mums was becoming more and more active. Its story is told in detail in Chapter 16, but prior to the public decision to terminate the AMP contract the Albany Mums were already starting to campaign on behalf of their beloved Practice. Having gained permission to attend a Maternity Services Liaison Committee (MSLC) meeting at King's on 26 November, 10 members of the group were able to ask questions about their concerns, and to challenge the statistics story as they saw it. MSLCs were multidisciplinary bodies which included lay people, practitioners, managers and commissioners. Their purpose was to meet regularly to improve local maternity care policy and practice, reflecting the findings of reliable evidence and parents' views. At this meeting, when asked about the recent closure of the home birth service and whether it might be possible to supervise or train the AMP midwives in this area of work, Leonie Penna reportedly commented (referring to the CMACE Report): *'Hopefully this report shows that there is* not only one thing that they are doing wrong *so retraining the Albany Midwives would not be an option'* (our emphasis). This was an extraordinary comment from someone who at that time was still officially the link obstetrician for the Practice. In response to this and other remarks made at that meeting, Pauline penned the following email to Leonie, demonstrating the Practice's frustration and upset:

> *'Your comments at the MSLC meeting, when a number of Albany mothers were present, were highly misleading and potentially defamatory. We hope that you will not repeat or publicise those comments to any third party in the future. Should it come to our attention that you have done so, we will not hesitate to seek legal redress. We invite you to make a formal apology forthwith.'*

No reply was received.

Closure meeting: 3rd December 2009

In the week following the MSLC meeting rumours that had been circulating came to a head. On Tuesday 1 December Sarah Dawson emailed requesting a meeting with the Practice, along with Katie and Leonie and Roland Sinker, Director of Operations. With everyone feeling pressurised, Pauline replied saying that the Practice was 'unable to make the meeting', was taking advice about how to respond to the CMACE Report, and needed in any case to see the proposed agenda. She also commented that 'in light of the comments made by Dr Penna (at the MSLC meeting), we do not feel it is appropriate for her to attend any proposed meeting between us and yourselves.' Tim Smart wrote the following day ignoring this, saying that a meeting had been set up and that Geraldine Walters (Director of Nursing and Midwifery) would also be in attendance. Late that evening Pauline wrote again confirming that the Practice would not be attending the meeting, but the following morning the pressure to meet continued. Roland Sinker phoned Pauline to say that King's was intending to terminate the contract and that 'it is necessary for us to come to a meeting this week, preferably today.' His concerns seemed to be about governance, saying that 'given the regulatory environment in which the Trust is operating, they have to be confident that services are appropriately governed.' He also confirmed that all 'outside contracts' were to be withdrawn. Feeling backed into a corner, Pauline sent a message to the recently established supporters' email group, saying:

> 'We have been told that if we do not attend a meeting this week we will be deemed to be in breach of contract and it will be terminated immediately. A group of midwives are therefore going to a meeting this afternoon to hear what is on the table so that we can have some time to consider our position. The time frame has just got a lot sharper!'

And so, exactly a year to the day from the very first shocking meeting, on the afternoon of Thursday 3 December 2009, members of the Practice went to a meeting at King's to hear their fate. Francine Allen from the RCM was present, as well as Roland Sinker and Geraldine Walters from King's management, and Katie Yiannouzis. As they had feared, the Practice members were told that the Trust had decided not to renew their contract, with definite termination of the contract at the end of March 2010.

Opening the meeting, Roland Sinker framed this momentous decision in terms of regulation, accountability, and governance. He discussed the Trust's accountability to the Board of Governors, their obligation to their insurers, and the need to satisfy the Care Quality Commission that the Trust's services were 'well governed'. He also hinted at fears around potential litigation claims. He then went on to say that the implication of this was that the Trust would not be renewing its contract with the Albany, nor with any other service with an 'arm's-length contract', and that this was a 'corporate decision'.

The midwives' hearts sank. They listened as Roland Sinker talked about the model of care that mattered so much to them, and that they knew in their hearts, and from their own evidence, was safe. 'Received letters... high standard of care... appreciated enormously... positive elements...'. These were empty words given what had just been announced. And yet there was an incredulous attempt to make it all sound caring: 'How can we look after you?' asked Roland Sinker. 'We want to take care of you,' said Geraldine Waters. 'We don't want to make it difficult,' said Katie Yiannouzis.

The midwives were reassured that they wouldn't be in financial difficulty, and that there would be no problem with pay up until the end of March, when the contract would end. But for the women in their caseload this would be the end of their Albany care, and they would be 'transitioned' into regular King's care as soon as possible. Two midwives from King's had already been allocated to take over the caseloads, and the handover would take place the following week.

As for the midwives in the Practice, Katie talked about jobs being available for them in the hospital: 'We want to transition you into King's.' In a letter to the Practice the following day summarising the outcome of the meeting, Roland Sinker stated the following, for 'the partners of the Practice who are midwives':

> 'You are invited to express an interest in working as a band 6 hospital midwife by 18th December 2009. If you tell us you want to work at King's you will be slotted into a vacant hospital midwife post from 1st January 2010...'

Unbelievably, these midwives, who collectively were considered by King's to be too dangerous to practise, were nevertheless individually being offered jobs within the Trust.

The day after this meeting King's issued the following press statement:

'Earlier this year, King's asked the Centre for Maternal and Child Enquiries (CMACE) to investigate concerns we had about the higher than usual number of babies born with serious health problems to women being cared for by the Albany midwifery practice. While the report from CMACE reinforced our own view of the excellent relationships formed between the Albany midwives and their expectant mothers, it also highlighted some serious shortcomings in terms of noncompliance with Trust policies and risk management procedures, particularly during labour and with newborn babies. We felt this was an unacceptable level of risk for our patients and were unhappy with the nature of the contractual arrangements. Therefore a decision has been taken to terminate our contract with Albany. We are committed to midwifery-led care for women, and believe strongly in giving women the right to choose a home-birth, which is why we have one of the highest home-birth rates in the country. Our approach will not change in this regard. We plan to establish a new midwifery practice using the same model we use for our other nine community midwifery practices – where the midwives are employed directly by King's and operate under much closer supervision. We value the personal qualities of the midwives working at the Albany, and have encouraged them to apply for midwifery jobs at King's. We would like to reassure patients that this decision has been taken with their safety and well-being in mind. We would also like to thank them for their patience as alternative arrangements for a small number of expectant mothers are being made.'

King's was repeating its view that it was not the individual midwives who were dangerous, but instead the Albany Practice model itself. The midwives could continue to work, provided they were employed and managed by the Trust. But the world-renowned, gold-standard, nationally and internationally recognised Albany Midwifery Practice, loved by the women and families it served, and a model for future midwifery, was to be closed.

Caroline Flint
Midwife

What did the closure of the Albany Practice mean to me, mean to us? The loss of hope, the loss of a future, the destruction of our professional *raison d'être*.

The Albany was what the research showed was the most successful form of midwifery care – where midwives formed a relationship with women and women formed a relationship with midwives. The midwives were autonomous, their practice was safe and calm. With their policy of suggesting to women that they didn't need to decide where to actually give birth until they were in labour and were experiencing what their labour was like, a high number of women gave birth at home. In 2008 49.5% of the women gave birth at home. Just think of the cost saving that represents. Half of the women did not use a hospital bed, hospital sheets, theatre, sutures, medications, staff, food, paper work, computer time, anaesthesia. This was a very cheap way of caring for women at the same time as being a much higher quality of care, and women were less traumatised by the birth experience. In fact much the opposite – women revelled in their birth experiences, feeling empowered and strong, managing breastfeeding much more easily, and entering motherhood confidently.

This was a joyous practice of midwifery. We saw it as the future of our profession. Where we would all end up when we grew up.

That was the problem – it was too successful. It showed up the mediocrity of normal maternity care, and as ever other midwives and obstetricians would 'speak up' on behalf of other women, saying 'It isn't fair that these women get better care.' And as usual, instead of transforming all care to be this way, the goose that laid the golden eggs was slaughtered. Mindless, stupid, blinkered, tragic and cruel.

This book will go a long way to helping the midwifery profession see what is needed. The figures will stand on their own showing us what we should be doing, how we should be practising, how we can truly be 'with woman'.

15
Fallout

'The closure of the service to me represented a kind of vandalism.'
Professor Lesley Page

In the weeks following the decision to terminate the Albany contract the whole Practice was in a state of shock and grief. The looming inevitability had become a devastating reality. Many tears were shed in sadness at what was lost and anger at the injustice of what had happened.

The midwives and Pauline were not just losing their jobs: they were watching helplessly as their philosophy of midwifery care was destroyed. But they needed to focus on all the women who were booked with them and to whom they could no longer offer care. A 'transition plan' was put in place, involving transfer of care from the AMP to just two King's midwives, who had been allocated to come to the Practice the following week to 'undertake a handover'. The Albany midwives knew straight away that this would lead to compromised care for the women involved.

In mid-December Tim Smart wrote in a letter to Beverley Beech:

> 'I would like to reassure you that the Trust is making every effort to ensure that mothers currently looked after by the Albany Practice have a smooth transition to the midwifery service of their choice, including the personal choice of home birth through one of the King's community midwifery practices.'

It soon became abundantly clear that simply stepping in and allocating two midwives was not going to provide the 'smooth transition' that Tim Smart had promised. Continuity of carer was being completely removed, and the women were upset, angry, and in some cases scared. In a tearful interview filmed by the *Guardian* a few days after the closure was announced, one of the mothers, who had had a previous positive birth with the Albany midwives, said:

> *'I'm due in six weeks and I'm suddenly not looking forward to it…*
> *it's a really horrible thing to think about [when you're] having a*
> *baby, but right now I'm dreading it.'*

The midwives were feeling powerless, and of course upset and concerned for the women whose care was being transferred, sometimes very late in their pregnancy. However, still determined to state their case and keep their heads held high, the AMP got back in touch with Eleena, the barrister who had supported them the month before. They felt they needed her input when responding to the termination letter from King's, in which it was stated that 'the Trust has decided to terminate the current contract on 22nd December 2009'. With Eleena's help, Pauline composed a letter to Roland Sinker at King's questioning the legal basis on which the termination decision was founded:

> *'Please could you confirm which clause in the contract you are*
> *invoking in respect of the early termination… The Practice was not*
> *given any opportunity to remedy any perceived breach (which we*
> *deny)… Further, we note that you would be the person responsible*
> *for resolving a dispute according to the arbitration clause in the*
> *contract, but have simply terminated the contract.'*

The AMP also felt it important to state its rejection of the safety allegations that had been dogging them for the whole of the previous year:

> *'You state that you no longer wish to contract care from the*
> *Albany Midwifery Practice, and that you have "very serious safety*
> *concerns" with our care. Whilst we are saddened by the decision*
> *in respect of the former, you are aware that we firmly dispute the*
> *basis for the latter.'*

In her letter, Pauline powerfully states that 'we have been somewhat blindsided by the decision', and asks for time to 'inform and consult with' those members of the Practice who were not partners (i.e. those who were not midwives). As for the partners, the message is very clear:

> 'None of the partners of the practice wishes to apply for a job with the Trust. This is because trust and confidence is now damaged beyond repair.'

The decision to close down the Albany Practice was undeniably final on the part of King's. Perhaps not surprisingly, given its reputation as a forward-looking, gold-standard service for women, the news of the closure sent shockwaves through the birthing community. Ongoing support for the Practice and the model of care is discussed elsewhere (see chapters 16 to 18), but there was also immediate support, both from within the midwifery world itself and from maternity campaigning organisations. Within four days AIMS had produced a press release entitled:

'SAFETY OF DISADVANTAGED WOMEN AND BABIES IS THREATENED BY KING'S CLOSURE OF THE ALBANY MIDWIFERY PRACTICE'

The press release stated: 'It is unacceptable to withdraw such a safe and much needed service from the poorest women in society.' Two days later the NCT released a press statement, saying 'the abrupt closure of the Albany Practice's vital service is extremely worrying for local women who value its service', and calling for 'a full independent inquiry into the maternity services of King's College Hospital NHS Foundation Trust, as a matter of urgency, using a study methodology which lends itself to meaningful statistical analysis.'

The closure of the Albany Practice made news headlines both locally and nationally. Coverage included articles in local papers in south-east London, as well as in the *Guardian*, and later on in a more reflective piece in *The Times*. There was also TV and radio coverage, with reports on More 4 News, BBC News, and the BBC London *Breakfast Show*. The *Guardian* online published a video highlighting a demonstration on the steps of King's, which contained moving interviews with some of the Albany Mums.

For the midwives, on the receiving end of King's' failures over the course of a long year, their mental health had been truly challenged. The continued questioning of their practice had taken its toll. Pauline commented: 'It was devastating for everyone but such a blow to midwifery confidence, and also desire to even be a midwife after such abuse. They were battered.'

Mary talked later about the complete lack of support and how damaging this was. She felt it undermined her confidence as a midwife, admitting to feelings of anxiety: 'I do think I have some aspects of post-traumatic stress from it'.

Understandably, none of the midwives wanted to take up the offer from King's of a job in the hospital. They had been part of an outstanding model of care and couldn't at the time imagine working differently. Years later, one of the midwives, Danielle, said:

> 'Working with strong, supportive and like-minded midwives and providing true continuity of care for inspirational women through their pregnancy and birth journey got me out of bed with a spring in my step every day. This was true midwifery and I don't think I've ever felt like a "proper" midwife since.'

Inevitably the impact of the closure of a service that had offered skilled, relationship-based continuity of care began to show in subsequent birth outcomes. The Albany Practice midwives collected outcome data for the women they had booked who were due to give birth in the next couple of months, and who were cared for in labour by other midwives. The numbers were small (21 women), but showed unexpectedly high intervention rates, with an increase in caesarean sections and instrumental

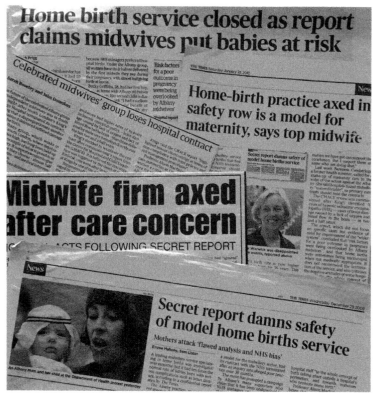

The closure in the news

births, and only one home birth. Three years earlier Jill Demilew had showed in her important report *Tackling Health Inequality: Supporting Wellbeing* that with a home birth rate in 2006 of 44.8 per cent, the Albany was contributing to King's' much-lauded overall home birth rate. Tim Smart, responding to a letter from the Albany Mums on 23 December 2009, said: 'The Trust runs nine other midwife-led community practices, who offer choice to the women of SE London, and at 9%, King's has one of the best rates of home birth in the UK.' However, by the summer of 2010 the home birth rate had dropped to an average of 5.4 per cent. The caesarean section rate had risen to 26.6 per cent from 22.1 per cent in 2006.

The loss of the Albany was also felt in other ways. Mary Newburn, researcher and birth activist, said:

> 'The loss of the Albany was huge for the families affected and the local community. It was devastating for the midwives who had invested so much and created something unique within the NHS. And for maternity charities and influencers it was a huge setback.'

All the members of the Albany Practice felt the closure keenly and personally. Somehow during those dark days at the end of 2009 they made themselves carry on, challenging where they could and turning their thoughts towards campaigning. They kept the women they had recently cared for in their minds, and at Christmas they organised a party for all the women and families to celebrate the good things they knew they had achieved.

Luke Zander

GP obstetrician and founder of the Forum on Maternity and the Newborn at the Royal Society of Medicine

The Albany Midwifery Practice is a name that is widely known and heralded in the field of midwifery for the nature of the care it provided. It represented a form of woman-centred midwifery care all too rarely achieved for both women and the professionals looking after them, which demonstrated a truly holistic approach to the management of pregnancy and birth for women and their families.

Much thought and debate is being devoted to the difficult question of how our maternity services can best be provided. Pregnancy and birth are fundamental human events with the potential for long-term life-enhancing repercussions, and the medical model of measuring success by the yardstick of the cemetery is not in itself adequate to take account of the dimensions that need to be satisfied. This is not in any way to suggest that mortality measurement is not of critical importance, but rather to stress the relevance of other factors.

As a GP working for over 30 years in close proximity to the deprived neighbourhood of south-east London in which the Albany Midwifery Practice was situated, I experienced at close hand, and came to greatly value and appreciate, the dedicated service that it provided for its community. Having a clinical and academic special interest in the delivery of community-based maternity services, and with a long-standing personal clinical involvement in the provision of care for women choosing to have a home birth, I became very aware of the nature and quality of the care provided by the AMP and the very high regard in which it was held.

The closure of the AMP, by the authority charged with the responsibility of providing optimal maternity services for its community, understandably caused deep distress and resentment within the locality, and much concern was expressed about the rationale and validity of the decision taken, not just locally but also nationally and even internationally, because of its perceived implications.

The closure caused many fundamental questions to be asked, and raised wide issues of general relevance to the current discussions taking place about the delivery of midwifery-based care. In 2010 I convened the Albany Model Advisory Group (AMAG), which met intermittently over three years. The members of the group, many of whom were in senior positions in their own fields of activity, acted in a purely personal and non-representative capacity. They were all exceedingly committed, and clearly felt that the importance of the issues raised by the action taken against the Albany warranted such a prolonged period of engagement. As well as the Albany practice manager, Pauline Armstrong, other members of AMAG were Debbie Chippington Derrick, Sarah Davies, Dr Nadine Edwards, Professor Mavis Kirkham, Professor Alison Mcfarlane, Dr Jo Murphy-Lawless, Mary Newburn, Professor Jane Sandall, Professor Cathy Warwick and myself.

The objective of the venture was to facilitate the exchange

of information and the development of ideas which could then be taken further through AMAG's support, and also to be of assistance to members in their own fields of activity. The many issues considered were not only to have some direct relationship to the actions taken against the Albany, but also to be of general relevance to other settings and situations.

I would like to take this opportunity to express my gratitude to those who generously gave of their time to participate in this attempt to achieve something of value through the collective consideration of different facets of the Albany saga, for the benefit of midwifery-led care in the future.

16

The community fights back

'You want to know what we want? What we want is what you took away.' Albany dad

Once the accusations about the Albany Midwifery Practice and its threatened and subsequent closure became public knowledge, a train of events was set in motion. The attack on the Albany Midwifery Practice touched a collective community nerve, and ignited a series of parallel and overlapping campaigns involving parents, activists, childbirth organisations, health practitioners and academics across the country. Of these, the story of the Albany Mums campaign is perhaps the most remarkable. A diverse and challenged community, unused to campaigning, drew on its outrage and determination to take on the upper echelons of power head on, usually with babies and toddlers in slings and buggies. It was an extraordinary effort.

The parents served by the Albany midwives were initially hampered by not knowing about the accusations against or investigations into the Albany Midwifery Practice. While the midwives had lived through nine months of investigations, these parents had had no inkling of the seriousness of the threat to their midwives until just weeks before the home birth service was suddenly suspended.

In September 2009 a few of the women who had most recently booked with the Albany Midwives became aware that something was seriously amiss. While they didn't know exactly what was going on, they knew that questions were being asked about the safety of their care and began to feel a deep sense of unease. One of the women remembers being told that King's now believed that 'this way of giving birth was unsafe'. What exactly did they mean by 'this way'? Emma Beamish, who became one of the leaders of the parents' campaign, was so concerned about the situation that she started weekly support meetings in her home near Peckham Pulse:

> 'it became kind of weekly. You know, on Wednesday after two o'clock, come round to Emma's house, and you never knew what state it might be in but the sofas were full and it certainly wasn't formal. I think we were wondering what we could do to help'.

The mothers who'd been meeting informally soon realised that their service really was under threat. Home births were being stopped, and one of their midwives was being suspended from practice. Upset and angry, they formed a campaign group called the Albany Mums. They set up a Facebook page that immediately attracted 700 followers, an extraordinary number for that time. They also started a petition, citing the Albany Midwifery Practice's excellent outcomes and saying: 'we call for these services for women and babies [...] to be reinstated forthwith'. This petition was signed by 4,000 people. The community knew from the start that families stood to lose something vital to their sense of agency and wellbeing. The Albany Mums were particularly concerned about the women whose babies were due soon and who were planning a home birth, as these women would now have to decide between a hospital birth with their Albany midwives or a home birth with a stranger.

Within weeks, the Albany Mums' outrage and distress intensified when they learned that their Practice was being closed with immediate effect. The newly formed Albany Mums group continued to grow and attract others who'd previously been looked after by Albany midwives and who wanted to support the campaign. There was a shared understanding that the service was special and offered families in Peckham something unique, and that in closing it King's was committing a serious injustice to the community, most especially to the women booked with the Albany midwives at the time. The group was diverse and most members had no direct experience of activism and were neither 'seasoned campaigners... nor revolutionary', but they felt passionate about saving their precious midwifery service. Their meetings continued to be a regular event, attended by:

> 'women who have almost nothing in common except that they happen to be mothers and they happen to have had Albany midwives... there are women with very little English, there are women from all different cultures and backgrounds'.

As one of the mums poignantly remarked:

> 'You know, this area has a lot of problems and it needs more help not less, and I just think it's a travesty... It just seems such a travesty to me that you would mess that up [by closing the Albany Practice] when everything else needs looking at round here'.

One of the Albany Mums, who happened to be a women's health campaigner, explained that the Albany model was rooted in a history of campaigns for better birth. She, like others, understood the health, wellbeing and safety benefits of trusting relationships between women and midwives. She said:

> 'and it was like to have that suddenly shut felt just outrageous... we were really outraged because of the dishonesty of the fact that they used health and safety which we knew was a nonsense, so it became like a howl of disbelief and injustice because this beautiful thing was not only being shut but it was wrongly accused and THAT was just one step too far'.

The injustice was keenly felt throughout the community. Whenever the Albany Mums talked to people in their locality about the closure of the Practice, there was the same disbelief and outrage. Families remembered their midwives with gratitude and love. One Albany Mum said: 'every person I've met in the wider community is grieving the loss of this model.' Another remarked, 'I miss the team and a big hole has been left in Southwark's healthcare service with the termination of the Albany', while a third said 'I don't think King's knows what it has started.' Despite the levels of poverty and other challenges, and the general disinclination to become involved in campaigns or donate to them, when the Albany Mums took to the streets to collect money for their campaign, the people of Peckham chipped in and many asked what they could do to help.

The Albany Mums felt they were very much 'learning as we went' as they'd 'never marched down the street for anything before... This wasn't a natural thing for us to be doing at all'. But they sought out help and advice wherever they could, and quickly learned where they might take their grievances and exert pressure on King's to reinstate their midwifery practice.

One of the Mums' first actions was to go to local MP Harriet Harman's surgery in October 2009, where they discovered that constituents were required to discuss their concerns first with the MP's councillors. The MP would then decide whether or not to take up the issue. Emma recalls that while talking to the councillor, the Mums felt listened to for the first time. They followed up the meeting with a letter to the councillor detailing their concerns, but incredibly never heard from her again. They visited and wrote to Harriet Harman's office repeatedly but to no avail. Months later they had still heard nothing. Finally, the Mums received a reply claiming rather unbelievably that their letter of complaint about the closure of the AMP had been dropped behind a filing cabinet. Harriet Harman did eventually send a letter to King's on behalf of the Mums on 8 March 2010. King's response on 24 March reiterated that its concerns were about safety. It blamed the midwives for being 'non-cooperative', showing neither insight nor 'willingness to work with the Trust to ensure the safety of the practice'. Harriet Harman acknowledged that the Albany Mums would be 'disappointed' but accepted that King's would not reconsider its decision to close the AMP. Instead she asked King's 'to meet with supporters of the Albany Practice and work together to develop future services'. But as events unfolded, the Mums felt that their input was unwelcome, ignored or avoided whenever possible. The Mums tried to set up a meeting with Harriet Harman in Parliament, but were told that there were more pressing issues for her to deal with than their concerns about the AMP closure, and that she had every faith in King's maternity services and could see no reason to probe any further. The Mums tried again but never heard anything more. It remains a mystery to them, to this day, that their MP, at the time the Minister for Women's Equal Opportunities, failed to engage with them or support them.

Following the suspension of the home birth service at the end of September 2009, the Mums asked if they could attend the next Maternity Services Liaison Committee (MSLC) meeting, so that they could ask questions about the suspension, the rumours about the possible closure of the Practice, the data on which this was based and to state their case to retain the AMP.

As mentioned in Chapter 14, the Albany Mums were given permission to attend an MSLC meeting on 26 November, and 10 Mums were present at the meeting that day. Emma recalls, however, that in a 'weird disconnect' the MSLC knew nothing about the suspension of the Albany home birth service. A discussion did take place, but, as recorded in the meeting minutes, each of the Mums' concerns was dealt with in the same way that the Albany midwives' questions had been. The same arguments were used: Albany babies were 10 times more likely to be admitted to the Special Care Baby Unit with HIE than other King's babies. No supporting evidence was provided, but Leonie Penna insisted that these were the 'facts'. The Mums asked questions about the CMACE Report and requested a copy of it. They were told that once the report had been checked by the Trust, it was for the Trust and the Albany Midwives only. When the Mums remained unconvinced by some of the replies, Leonie brought the discussion to a close by saying that Katie Yiannouzis had offered to meet the Albany Mums to discuss any further questions.

The day after that meeting the Mums wrote to Tim Smart expressing their deep concern about the investigations into the AMP. They enclosed a bundle of letters of support for the Practice from Albany families. They received no response. Following the decision to close the Practice on 3 December, Emma wrote to Tim Smart again on 15 December, this time specifically asking about replacement services for the women. Eventually, on 23 December, Tim Smart replied to their original letter with the now standard King's narrative that although the Practice was liked by women, and achieved high breastfeeding rates and low mortality rates for babies, the HIE rate was significantly higher than for the rest of King's babies.

Five Albany Mums attended the next MSLC meeting at the end of January 2010. They were very surprised to learn that the MSLC had not been consulted or even informed about the closure of the AMP. They were extremely disappointed and frustrated that Leonie Penna, Katie Yiannouzis and a King's manager who could have answered their questions about the closure and the CMACE Report had sent their apologies to the meeting. As the Albany Mums had been tabled on the agenda, they felt that this was 'an open attempt to avoid answering all the questions that have arisen since the previous meeting'.

The Mums were not sent an invitation to the next meeting in April, despite having provided their email addresses. They learned afterwards that a report had been given to the MSLC members claiming that all was going well in Peckham, with two community midwives now practising there, and that women there no longer wanted home births. Without the Mums present, there was no one to contradict this, or to tell the MSLC that women were struggling to get maternity care and that proper provision had not been made. No one was able to ask when a replacement service would be up and running. In the event, a replacement service had still not materialised over two years later. Following this meeting, and wanting to ensure that the Albany Mums' voices continued to be heard, Emma asked to become a full member of the MSLC.

Emma usually attended the meetings on her own. Many of the other Albany Mums found it difficult to attend, as they were either working at the time of the meetings or needed to pick up children from school or nursery. The requirement to submit names prior to the meeting was an additional barrier 'because people didn't know if they could come or not' until the last minute. Many of the Mums also found the board room at King's intimidating and difficult to access. And as if this wasn't enough, the Albany Mums were asked to submit topics for the agenda well ahead of the meeting. While all of this was normal practice for those working at King's, for the Mums it made contributing to the meetings almost impossible. Emma dreaded the meetings, and said 'it took a lot to go'. However, she felt compelled to continue to represent the Albany parents and remind the MSLC members about what their community had lost and what it now needed from midwifery services.

Reflecting later, the Albany Mums felt that they were tolerated at the MSLC meetings 'to make it seem as if we were being listened to'. They recalled being repeatedly told that they didn't know the full story: 'You don't have all the information, if only you knew what we knew, you wouldn't be supporting these midwives. Take it from us, as professionals, they're dangerous'. The inference was that 'you'll look stupid' once things were revealed. As the Albany Mums continued to ask awkward questions, senior clinicians and managers stopped attending the MSLC meetings. Feeling very disheartened, the Mums concluded that the MSLC could be of no help to them.

Despite the challenges they faced, the Mums lost no time in staging demonstrations and contacting the press. Their creativity and persistence knew no bounds. Within two days of the decision to close the Practice they organised a protest attended by 200 people, having 'begged and borrowed' funds to make T-shirts and baby vests for the event. They refused to be diverted to the park behind the hospital where a demonstration would have been

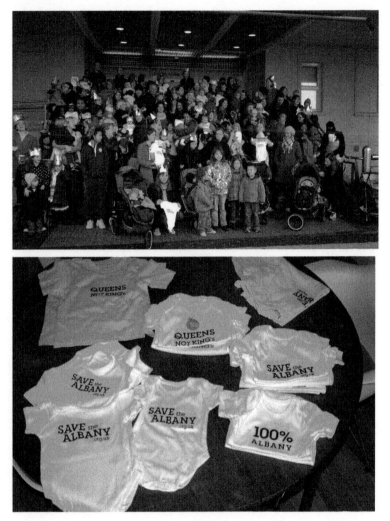

Above: *Albany parents and others demonstrate on the steps of King's*
Below: *Baby T-shirts and vests for the demonstration*

invisible, instead gathering on the main steps of King's College Hospital.

The peaceful protest comprised mainly Albany Mums and their families, holding homemade placards. Even though they were careful not to block entrances or exits or cause any difficulties for

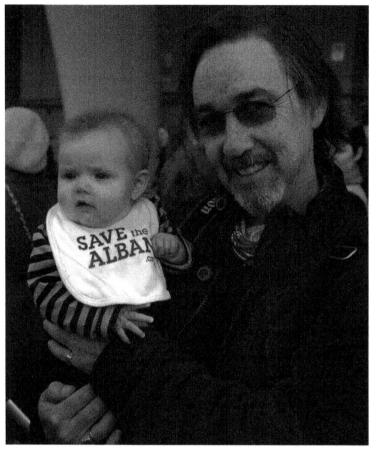

An Albany dad and baby at the demonstration

the hospital, they were told by officials that they had created an obstruction and posed a danger. As one of the organisers, Emma was told that in the future she would not be allowed onto King's premises. She felt that this threat was designed to intimidate her, with the intention of undermining the campaign and ridding the hospital management of the annoyance and embarrassment that it was causing King's.

The protest achieved media coverage and was reported online by the *Guardian* in a video later that day. There were emotional interviews with some of the Albany Mums, one of whom said 'we have to fight for this really, not just for the women of Peckham but this is the model that should be spread out across the country' and another said 'these women are offering a service that's literally like a light... a light in a very dark place'.

Despite the setbacks, the Albany Mums pressed on. They contacted the Care Quality Commission (CQC). The CQC had been set up on 1 October 2008 as an independent regulator of NHS services to 'make sure health and social care services provide people with safe, effective, compassionate, high-quality care'. It had powers to hold health services to account and could even prosecute for inflicted harms. It stated on its website that it wished to hear from and would act on the public's experiences and views. It specifically invited contact from any member of the public who had any concerns about a local health service and stated that one of its roles was to 'protect the rights of vulnerable people'. This seemed exactly what the Mums were looking for. They had grave concerns about a local service, their community was definitely vulnerable and they needed someone with some authority to listen to them and act on their behalf. Maybe something could be done.

The Mums sent a letter to the CQC on 14 December 2009, expressing their concerns about the loss of their midwifery practice, the lack of provision for women who had been booked with the Practice midwives, 'the absolute lack of response from the Trust' and its failure to engage with them despite their efforts, their serious doubts about the CMACE Report, and their call for 'an open and truly independent investigation into the maternity services throughout King's Hospital Foundation Trust'.

The Mums experienced the same disappointing lack of response that they had encountered from the Trust and their MP. Juggling babies, families and work, Emma or another mum phoned the CQC repeatedly, but they were always told to phone back at different times to speak to the appropriate person. They could never get through to the 'right' person, 'the administration was enormous and just having to ring and be tenacious and trying to get someone's name and ring again...' was immensely demanding.

A few days before Christmas, the seemingly tireless Albany Mums staged a nativity scene outside the Department of Health in London, to demand that their service be reinstated and to request a copy of the CMACE Report that King's had refused to send them. The Mums, dads, children and supporters dressed up as angels, kings and shepherds and sang well-known Christmas carols with their own campaigning words composed by Albany mum Rix Pyke (see Appendix 2). As one of the Mums told a reporter at the scene:

> *'This is a cover up. If the reasons for closing this practice are really health issues, and not politically motivated, why can't we see the report? We want a public enquiry so that the truth can be told.'*

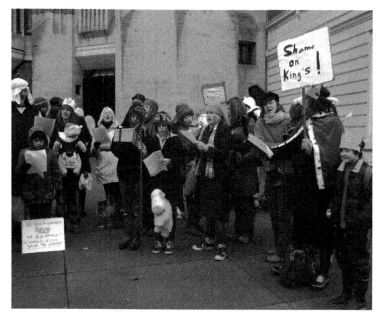

Singing at the demonstration outside the Department of Health

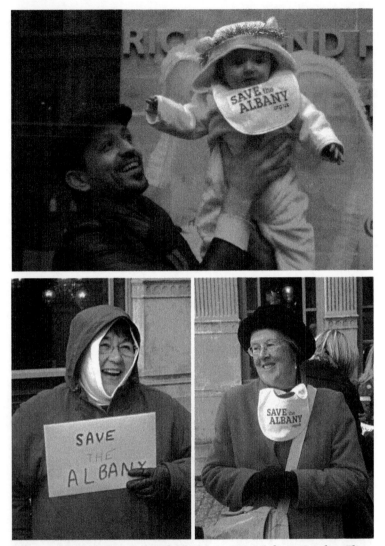

Above: *Albany baby angel at the demonstration* Below: *Caroline Flint and Beverley Beech at the demonstration*

In the run up to Christmas a series of articles was published in the media, with the story of the Albany closure being covered both in the local and national press. *The Times* online quoted the Mums saying that the CMACE Report was 'a flawed analysis that had been withheld from the public.' Baroness Cumberlege called for 'greater transparency over the termination' of the AMP contract and said that 'it is essential that the report should be made public'. Another piece in *The Times* quoted one of the Mums saying that the Albany Practice had been closed 'under a shroud of secrecy and without any public justification'.

The Mums continued to contact senior managers at the Trust and on 25 February 2010 four Mums and their babies attended a meeting with Katie Yiannouzis, Sarah Dawson and Kate Brintworth from King's, and a representative from the local Primary Care Trust (PCT). The Mums had a list of questions that they had been trying to get answers to for months, but were given only an hour to discuss them. Their main concerns were the securing of a short-term replacement service for the women who had lost their Albany midwives, as there was still no reliable midwifery service in Peckham nearly three months after the closure. They also wanted to ask about plans for the future of their midwifery services, and how and when King's proposed to carry out its promised consultation with their community. They questioned the data used by King's to close the Practice, and reasserted their conviction that the AMP was safe, but were told that the Practice's data was flawed, and that the midwives' care had become unsafe. The Mums were told that the Trust would not be removing the statement on its website, which stated that it had closed the Practice on the grounds of safety. When challenged further, Katie told them that the midwives were still 'disputing the figures' and that they 'had total lack of insight into their own practice'. She claimed that if they had just accepted the King's figures 'there would still be an Albany Practice'.

The Mums were then invited to describe the kind of midwifery service they wanted. When they said that they wanted caseload midwifery, as practised by the Albany Midwives, they were told that this wasn't possible, and that other midwifery services that were not case-loading were evaluated by women just as positively as the Albany Practice had been. Emma described King's' refusal to engage with what the Mums wanted as a consistent theme: it was a 'no to everything [...] that's just not possible, you know, you won't know your midwife, you can't have access to your midwife, you can't have a drop-in centre, that's not how it works – but these are what we want'. The heartbreaking quote from an Albany dad at the start of this chapter captures the feeling of injustice: 'You want to know what we want? What we want is what you took away'. A disadvantaged community defined its own needs for maternity care, was ignored and had its needs redefined by external organisations supposedly there to serve it.

One of the main arguments used by King's managers was the introduction of the European Working Time Directive, which had come into effect in 2004 to ensure a safer and healthier working environment and better conditions for workers. Practitioners were no longer allowed to work the long hours that they had been working in the past, a particularly important advance for junior doctors. This had not previously been raised in relation to the AMP and the Mums knew that this was not a plausible argument against case-loading midwifery. As long as the midwives had a contract in which they could manage their own time they were able to work within the European Working Time Directive. However, the idea of the midwives managing their own time had clearly become unacceptable for a Trust that preferred to employ midwives directly and have control over their time and their work, making it possible to redeploy them at a moment's notice to wherever it was felt they were needed in the service.

The arguments went back and forth and then moved to why a public consultation had not taken place before the closure of the Practice. The Mums knew that there was a statutory duty on Trusts to carry out a public consultation about any significant change to the provision of health services within their jurisdiction. The PCT representative replied that King's 'didn't feel it was significant enough to warrant a formal consultation'. Given the uniqueness of the Albany Midwifery Practice and the health benefits it brought to a community considered to be severely disadvantaged, it was difficult to comprehend this dereliction of duty.

In response to pressure from the Mums, King's eventually put together a consultation about what kind of midwifery services were wanted by their wider community. This was a disappointingly superficial tick-box exercise designed to show that women did not particularly want caseload midwifery and were content with their current midwifery care. The questionnaire was distributed to women in the locality, but the Mums quickly realised that copies had not been sent to women previously looked after by the AMP. A member of the CQC visited to check that the consultation was being properly carried out, so the Mums informed her that they had been excluded from the exercise and asked her why. Again they heard nothing back from her or the CQC.

The Mums pressed King's on this and in the end it was agreed that Albany mothers be included in the consultation. However, the electronic questionnaire was difficult to access in the community: 'our local population is very, very poor in general, so finding parents that have access to the internet and have a computer at home is [difficult]... so we had to battle for paper questionnaires'. Having achieved this, the Mums were then expected to distribute the questionnaires, as well as collect and return them. Miraculously, they managed to do this but they 'never heard another word' about it. All in all, the Mums felt that this was yet another way in which the Trust had failed to engage with them and what their community needed, while at the same time making it look as if it had.

The Albany Mums then turned to their local Primary Care Trust. PCTs were set up in 2001, and replaced by Care Commissioning Groups (CCGs) in April 2013. Until then, they were responsible for 'commissioning primary, community and secondary health services from providers'. The Mums were beginning to wonder whether the PCT would be able to directly commission the Albany Midwifery Practice, as King's seemed either unwilling or unable to replicate the Practice in Peckham. They requested a public meeting, which took place on 28 April. Around 30 Albany parents attended, as well as members of the Southwark PCT and managers and senior midwives from King's. Having been ignored and silenced for so long, the frustration and anger of the parents at having such a valuable service taken away from them spilled out at the meeting. Emma could see straight away that a similar meeting would never happen again, but explained, 'you know, that is what engagement looks like'. Yet again, the parents were told that they didn't know enough and that King's was keeping them safe. The parents refused to accept this and demanded their midwifery service back. In response, they were told that they were 'selfish' and 'unreasonable' to want the kind of midwifery care that they had previously had because this was 'detrimental to the welfare of midwives', and would take resources and experienced midwives away from other local areas. The parents were accused of being angry, swearing and being too difficult to work with. After the meeting they were told, as Emma predicted, that the PCT would not meet with them again, and she commented 'the truth is that some parents raised their voices, but nobody swore. They were passionate and they were not being listened to'.

After all their efforts, the Mums were now feeling despondent and frustrated and described being up against the 'King's machine' and meeting 'brick walls' at every turn. They were also feeling the 'insidious' impact of being told repeatedly that everything being done was in their best interests, and 'you're not in full possession of the facts'. This eventually began to whittle away at their confidence. In essence, the campaigners had experienced the same lack of engagement that the Albany Midwives had encountered the previous year. Eventually, the Albany Mums 'ran out of juice really. I think we were *really* successfully stonewalled'.

The Mums' campaign laid bare the depth of power disparities between communities and some of the most powerful organisations and structures around them. When attempting to engage with King's, their MP, the local PCT and the CQC, the Albany Mums had been either ignored or side-lined. Senior members of the NCT or AIMS, for example, were more successful in reaching the relevant people and setting up meetings. But in the end no one could bring these bodies to account, not even organisations set up specifically with this aim, such as the MSLC and the Scrutiny Committees (see Chapter 18). The MSLC had no powers to compel senior managers to attend to answer the Mums' questions, and while the Scrutiny Committees could ask probing questions and provide recommendations, they had no powers to compel the Trust to act.

The campaign led by parents in Peckham showed stark democratic deficits within our society and how violence against a community can be enacted with impunity on those whose lives are negatively impacted by this. It also shows the resourcefulness, strength, determination, creativity and integrity of communities in the face of these seemingly immovable prejudices and 'monoliths'. Nonetheless, the impact of the campaign on some of the most active Mums added a layer of trauma that they still live with today. Their story is a testimony to the Albany families and their midwives in equal measure.

Serra
Albany mum to Laila and A'isha

Despite the inevitable concerns associated with a first pregnancy, one thing I knew for certain was that I wanted continuity of care for my daughter's birth. I naively thought that this was a given for women during pregnancy, so was surprised to discover that this was in fact, not the case. Therefore, being looked after by the Albany Practice in Peckham almost felt like I had won the lottery! A local practice, who offered everything I'd dreamed of for my pregnancy and birth. I don't take for granted how lucky I was. At the start of my pregnancy, I was nervous and apprehensive. However towards the end, after months of prenatal classes and talks with the amazing Albany midwives and my fellow Albany mums (and dads), I felt strangely confident and relaxed. I'm certain that my feelings are shared by many of those cared for by the Practice, which is why the closure was so poignant for so many of us in the community. The initial shock and disbelief at this terrible injustice soon turned to anger and a rousing sense of determination. As mothers, we felt compelled to stand up and support these women who'd given us so much, at a time when we were considered so vulnerable.

The Albany Midwives had instilled a sense of fearlessness in me that is hard to describe. Walking alongside these women during the 'Reclaiming Birth' march felt like the start of a revolution. It was in many respects. Too often, women's rights are ignored or deemed unimportant. We refused to accept that 'our' practice was dangerous and we were determined to fight the closure with everything we had. That space that the Albany midwives occupied in Peckham was a safe haven for me and so many others. A place where open and honest conversations were welcome and laughter and (happy) tears common. I'm so proud to be an Albany mum and will forever be grateful for the experience I had with the practice. My hope is that more women are able to have Albany type care and feel as empowered and respected as I did, to make the right choices for their pregnancy and birth.

17
A politician's support

In autumn 2009 Pauline attended a parliamentary focus group meeting organised by the Liberal Democrat Party. As the Practice manager, she had been invited to attend to represent the AMP at this meeting, which was looking at innovative issues in healthcare. She arrived early, as did Norman Lamb MP, who was the Liberal Democrats' health spokesman. The two of them got talking, and as Pauline later remarked, 'my enthusiasm for the Practice really sparked his interest.' Following the meeting Norman Lamb expressed a wish to visit the Practice in Peckham, but sadly the Practice was closed down before this could be arranged.

At the start of 2010, as the campaigns began to take shape, lists were drawn up of influential people who could be supportive and helpful. Norman Lamb was of course included. While other politicians were wary of getting involved, the closure of the Albany Practice seemed to strike a chord with this gentle and moral-minded politician. In March 2011, when the Albany midwives finally contacted Norman Lamb and sent him their response to the CMACE Report, he immediately saw the injustice of the situation, and replied saying that he was 'extremely concerned about a number of the issues that you identify'. He attached to his reply a letter that he had drafted to send to CMACE, with copies to go to the Department of Health, the Chief Executive at King's and the CQC. In the letter he stated:

> 'I was acutely aware of the very positive reports of the work of the Albany Midwifery Practice and the outcomes that they had apparently achieved during the period of operation, and I was very distressed to hear of its demise following the CMACE report. It seemed to me that something of enormous value had been lost and if it is the case that inaccuracies or work of insufficient

robustness had led to this project's demise, then that really is wholly unacceptable'.

Tim Smart, the Chief Executive at King's, sent an unsatisfactory response, in which he quoted the statement that King's had put on its website, referring to the 'safety record' of the Practice. Norman Lamb forwarded this to the AMP asking for a reaction. Pauline and Becky, by now working together in an effort to reinstate the reputation of the Practice, responded by thanking him for his interest and support, saying: 'We believe that this damning quote is impeding our ability to promote the Albany model of care.' Having clarified the inaccuracies in Tim Smart's response, they went on to say:

> 'Whilst we are not looking at reinstatement as a Practice, we are very keen to clear this model of care of any slur and be able to promote and celebrate this model of midwifery throughout the country and indeed the world... We have struggled to get anyone in authority to listen and can't emphasise enough how important your interest has been.'

In October Norman Lamb wrote back to Tim Smart, asking him for a full response to his earlier letter:

> 'Could you now deal with the concerns that they raise in their response to the CMACE Report? You will note that they make the point that the internal audit was challenged by two professional statisticians and they are concerned that it is still quoted on the King's website.
>
> I note that they make reference to your assertion that King's has set up a replacement group practice. I understand that this has not happened. Could you comment on this?
>
> I also note that during the first 10 years of the practice the perinatal mortality rate was half that of Southwark as a whole. Surely this is an excellent performance. Finally, I note that the inquest into the incident involving a newborn baby in September 2009 found no

evidence of neglect on the part of the midwife. I would welcome
your comments on this as well.

I remain extremely concerned about an apparently unfair slur on
this practice resulting in the loss of something which seemed to me
to be really valuable.'

An increasingly unsatisfactory correspondence between these
two men continued for the following year. Beverley Beech from
AIMS also wrote to Norman Lamb in October 2011, raising wider
questions about the state of the maternity services. In his reply
Norman Lamb said 'I have to say that I have been horrified by the
way in which the Albany Midwifery Practice was treated'.

In December 2011, Tim Smart, having failed to reply to the
questions raised in Norman Lamb's letter, wrote suggesting a
meeting 'to discuss the issues'. In his letter he suggested that
Simon Hughes (MP for the constituency of Bermondsey and Old
Southwark in London) join the meeting; indeed, he said that Simon
Hughes 'has also said that he would like to join this meeting'.
Norman Lamb forwarded this letter to Pauline and Becky, saying
that if the meeting were to take place he would be keen for them to
attend. They replied with a comprehensive letter, pointing out that
Tim Smart had failed to answer any of Norman Lamb's specific
questions, and that this should happen before any meeting took
place. They commented:

> *'The suggestion for a meeting without any clear indication of*
> *its purpose causes us considerable concern, due to our previous*
> *experience with King's management. During the long and sorry*
> *saga of the closure of the Albany Practice we had many meetings,*
> *sometimes called with very short notice and often with no agenda.*
> *We were subjected to what we can only describe as bullying during*
> *those meetings, with extra people brought in without our prior*
> *knowledge, and with our point of view seldom listened to.'*

Pauline and Becky were surprised and concerned about the

seemingly arbitrary suggestion that Simon Hughes join the meeting. They said:

> 'The relevance of the suggested involvement of Simon Hughes has no explanation in Tim Smart's letter and is not at all clear. King's College Hospital is not in Simon Hughes's constituency, nor is he the MP for the area served by the Albany Practice. We are therefore curious to know why Simon Hughes has "said that he would like to join this meeting", and indeed, how he would even know about it.'

Is it possible that Tim Smart was inviting one of his friends (or acquaintances) to support him in a difficult meeting with an MP who was asking questions he found difficult to answer?

In view of his obvious continued interest in the Albany story, Pauline and Becky decided that it would be useful to have a face-to-face meeting with Norman Lamb. This was arranged for 30 January 2012 at Portcullis House, part of the Parliamentary Estate, where MPs have their offices. A briefing was prepared explaining the background to the AMP and a timeline of events since December 2008. Pauline remembers that she felt 'quite important' that day; certainly it felt that somebody with a degree of authority, and hopefully influence, was taking the issue very seriously. Immediately following this meeting Norman Lamb wrote again to Tim Smart, thanking him for his offer of a meeting, and saying:

> 'I would certainly be keen to meet with you, but I would like representatives of the Albany Midwifery Practice to be present at that meeting so that the discussion can be fully informed of their perspective. However, before such a meeting takes place, I do feel that it is appropriate to have your written response to each of the points I set out in my letter of 20th October last year.'

In the letter Norman Lamb referred to the challenging of the internal audit and the CMACE Report by professional statisticians, and the fact that the disputed findings of the internal audit remained on the King's website. He said: 'the stain on the character of the practice and the model of care remains. This causes me great concern.' And astutely he commented:

> 'Finally, the point that I want to stress above all else is that those involved in the Albany Practice fully accept that this practice is gone – however tragic that is. What they want to ensure is that a model of care which is widely regarded in midwifery as extremely positive is not tainted by the CMACE Report and internal audit and what happened to the Albany Practice. It is therefore essential that the remaining slur is removed so that women elsewhere can benefit from a model of care which appears to have got such good outcomes.'

Backwards and forwards it went. Tim Smart replied to Norman Lamb's request for clarification, except that in his reply his facts were not correct. It seems that he was feeling more and more challenged, and possibly backed into a corner. He definitely did not like the idea of meeting with anyone from the AMP, saying: 'From the Trust's perspective, it would not be appropriate for members of the Albany Practice to attend.' He was also clearly not enjoying being held to account by a Member of Parliament. He agreed to a meeting, but tried to put a stop to the 'continuing exchange of correspondence'. When Norman Lamb wrote again in June asking Tim Smart to comment on the statisticians' critiques of King's internal audit, he refused, saying:

> 'In my previous letters, I have provided you with information to explain the rationale behind our decision which was taken in the best interests of women and babies. As I stated previously, King's internal audit was never designed as a statistical analysis; it simply flagged that the HIE rates for the Albany Practice were high compared to other parts of the maternity service and this triggered the need for an investigation. I therefore do not think it appropriate to provide a full response to the critiques you enclosed.'

Becky had seen an example of Tim Smart's refusal to continue with written correspondence in a difficult situation before. In early 2010, having discovered that she had been referred to the NMC, but with no information about the reasons for this (and with the Head of Midwifery refusing to respond to her letters), Becky had tried to pursue the matter with Tim Smart, but he had refused to enter into any further correspondence (see Chapter 20).

In September 2012 Norman Lamb became Minister of State for Health in the Conservative and Liberal Democrat coalition government. Becky and Pauline wrote to him the following month, saying: 'we feel greatly reassured that there is now a minister with a particular interest in maternity care. We realise of course that you will now be busier than ever, but we hope nevertheless that you will continue to pursue this very important matter.' Unfortunately, maternity services fell outside Norman Lamb's portfolio within the Department of Health, which limited his involvement. However, reflecting on the situation later, he felt sure that he would have wanted to ask further questions. But with Tim Smart refusing further correspondence, refusing to respond to reasonable requests for information, and refusing to allow an open and constructive meeting, it seemed that all possible avenues had been explored and found to be dead ends. There was nothing more that this committed MP could do.

Baroness Julia Cumberlege

In 1992 as a new government minister I was encouraged to take a subject that was of interest and to follow it through. My chosen subject was maternity services. Having given birth to three sons I had experience. Previously I had chaired the Brighton Health Authority and heard the stories of birthing women which made my toes curl – surely we could do better?

Having set up a panel to examine, advise, and listen to a wide range of people we produced our 1993 report *Changing Childbirth*.

In the various reports I have chaired I know it is important to go out and witness good practice, areas in which innovation drives services into better territories. It is always better if the users who are receiving the services tell you what they think and feel. Unlike some NHS services the maternity cohort is younger, often outspoken with strong opinions and conscious that they cannot afford an alternative to NHS provision. Giving birth is possibly the best, the most important and hardest experience they will ever encounter. Bringing forward and rearing the next generation is one of the greatest contributions we women can make to the future of a good and thriving society.

In our research for *Changing Childbirth* we learnt of the Albany Practice. Here was something unique, a different way of working with women and their families. Visiting the Albany I immediately sensed the joy of the midwives working with women. There were no precious attitudes, no grumbles, but a true sense of worth, knowing what they were doing was right for women and their babies. They were working in Peckham, in the Borough of Southwark in London, which was ranked at the time as the 14th most deprived district of 354 in England, and had the highest proportion of babies born with low birth weight. More than half of the women on the Albany's books were from Black, Asian and Minority Ethnic communities. It was a challenging place for any service in which to operate.

Having skilfully negotiated a contract with King's College Hospital Trust it was reasonable that King's should commission an independent evaluation of the Albany Practice. This showed that it had a higher home birth rate, a lower induction rate, a higher vaginal birth rate, a lower elective caesarean section rate and a very high level of continuity where 89% of women were attended during labour by their primary midwife and Albany midwives were in attendance at 98% of the births. Various qualitative studies also commented on the positive experiences for women associated with the relationship that continuity of carer provided.

Spurious allegations were made on safety grounds, but none were proven. The NHS finds it hard to accept competitors, however small, which prove there are better ways to care for women, their babies, and their families.

In 2009 the Albany Midwifery Practice was closed. This was a tragedy for the passionate midwives, and a tragedy for the women who would have benefitted from a safer and more personal service in a deprived area.

When I was commissioned by Sir Simon (now Lord) Stevens to review maternity services for England in the 2016 *Better Births* report, we built on what we had learnt from the Albany and other continuity of carer models. The difference between *Changing Childbirth* and *Better Births* was the work by the Cochrane Collaboration and other research organisations that proved without a doubt that this model of care provides a more acceptable service for women and their partners, and a safer service for mothers and their babies.

We should never forget when working with women and their families that this baby will never be born again, and this woman will never give birth to this baby again – it is a precious new beginning for mother and child. We should question unnecessary interventions which disrupt the birth experience for the mother and affect the wellbeing of her future child. We should seek to ensure relationship care, the relationship between the mother and her baby, the other parent and the baby, the baby and the family and also the relationship between women and midwives, women and their doctors and the relationship between all the members of the caregiving team. Relationship care is the child of continuity of carer and should be experienced by every expectant and birthing mother. Nationally we are making progress and know this is the best chance of success – it is our generation which must make the difference.

18
A wider issue

In early summer 2009, Nadine Edwards was collecting material for an AIMS *Journal* on inspiring, exemplary midwifery models of care that were working well in the UK. Although not closely acquainted with the Albany Midwifery Practice, she knew about its achievements and that it was held in very high regard by women, midwives and academics, so asked the Practice if it was possible to submit an article. She was delighted when the midwives said yes. Weeks passed and finally Pauline Armstrong, the Practice Manager, phoned to explain that the Practice was under investigation and that the midwives now felt unable to contribute to the *Journal*. This was the first that Nadine had heard about any threat to the Practice. She was extremely shocked and

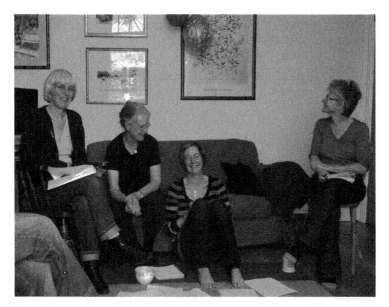

First campaign meeting with Margaret Jowitt, Mavis Kirkham,
Nadine Edwards and Sarah Davies

felt very strongly that something had to be done. The Albany Midwifery Practice was an iconic innovation in midwifery, and for it to be under threat seemed unthinkable. She asked Pauline and the midwives if they would allow her to set up a meeting to support the Practice. This was agreed and a date was set for 23 October.

The meeting in Becky's home brought together women from all over the UK, including Albany Mums, the Albany midwives and several members of AIMS and ARM, as well as some senior midwives and influential researchers. A packed agenda had been compiled, which included the Albany midwives telling their story and a discussion about what to do next.

The distress of the wider community was similar to that felt by the Albany Mums. At this first meeting an umbrella organisation, the Albany Action Group (AAG), was formed with the aim of protecting both the Practice and its model of care. The AAG attracted support from other childbirth organisations and individuals, and after the closure of the Practice it continued to meet in members' homes for eight years. The Group became a hub for those involved to discuss and plan strategy as the campaign evolved. As Pauline commented:

> 'The amount of work done by people – non-Albany – really is phenomenal. It shows how important the model is, and how women and midwives need to believe in something better.'

Professor Wendy Savage, a London obstetrician who had been a staunch advocate for women's reproductive decision-making, became a key supporter. She had been forced into a high-profile public enquiry in 1986 after her male obstetric colleagues trawled through her obstetric cases, cherry-picked several and accused her of dangerous practice. The *Guardian* noted that 'The suspension was seen as politically motivated, stemming from colleagues' hostility to her enthusiasm for community healthcare and home births rather than hi-tech hospital-based medicine'. Local women mounted a campaign to support her court case, which attracted a large following in the UK and abroad. Wendy told the story of her fight for justice in her book *The Savage Enquiry*. She clearly saw the parallels between her case and the Albany story, and having looked after the money remaining in her campaign fund for over 20 years, she donated this to the Albany Action Group.

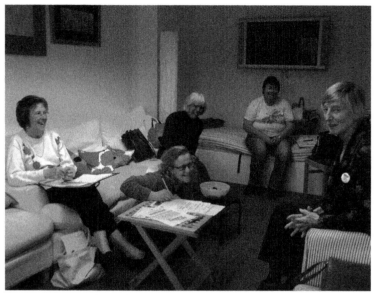

Members of the AAG with Wendy Savage (right)

The initial aims of the AAG were to persuade King's to remove the statement about the Albany Practice from its website, to clear the Practice's name, and to reinstate it. No stone was left unturned as the Action Group repeatedly contacted King's and its regulatory bodies, explored political avenues, sought out influential allies, contacted the press, wrote press releases and briefing papers, submitted Freedom of Information requests, organised demonstrations, became active on social media and attended countless meetings. The Action Group took every opportunity to call King's to account for closing a vital service.

It is no exaggeration to say that hundreds and hundreds of

letters and emails were sent on behalf of the Albany Midwifery Practice, detailing the Practice's excellent outcomes, critiquing the flawed statistics used to close the Practice, calling for King's maternity services as a whole to be evaluated and requesting that the statement on its website describing the Practice as unsafe be removed. Initially the Action Group members called for the reinstatement of the Practice. Later, they called for a similar midwifery service to replace the one that had been lost.

Letters and emails flooded in to King's. Many were directed to the Chief Executive, Tim Smart. Dr Mark Ashworth, as previously mentioned, wrote to him on 25 November 2009, urging King's to take 'note of the viewpoint of our general practice'. He referred to the very high standard of care provided by the midwives and pointed out that their work directly contributed to reducing health inequalities.

Many of those writing called for a full investigation into King's outcomes as a whole. They pointed out the flaws in the Case Series, the internal audit and the CMACE Report, and that none of these provided evidence that the AMP outcomes were poorer than those in other parts of King's maternity services, because King's statistics had not been examined and no comparison had been made. For example, the RCM stated that 'conclusions about safety cannot be drawn without further evaluation'. Alison Macfarlane and many others expressed similar sentiments. Wendy Savage wrote to the *Times* on 10 December 2009, concluding her letter with a quote from Sir Iain Chalmers (one of the founders of the Cochrane Collaboration) saying that 'it is wrong to accept opinion which is not based on evidence'.

Many commentators suggested that by accusing the Albany Midwives of dangerous practice with no reliable evidence, King's had done a great disservice to the community in Peckham, the Albany midwives and to midwifery in general. Denis Walsh, an Associate Professor of Midwifery, commented that the AMP closure had serious implications for the future of the profession. Sarah Davies, senior midwifery lecturer at Salford University, warned that, 'If King's is allowed to get away with this behaviour, midwifery will be massively weakened'.

The response from Tim Smart and other King's managers to any critiques or questions about the closure invariably attempted to justify their actions on the grounds of safety, as purportedly shown by their internal audit. Tim Smart had previously had a 30-year career in business (including with the oil company Shell, and British Telecom) and admitted to the NCT in a phone call that he had no scientific background, that he had to be seen to take action, and that he had been told that if he failed to do anything about the AMP he would be to blame.

King's Hospital Trust was clearly more open to meeting with a national organisation than with local parents. The NCT managed to secure meetings with various managers at King's, as well as with Tim Smart, in December 2009 and January 2010. It deduced that the closure was due to 'a management failure – which may have (or more likely has not) led to a safety issue', but was unable to persuade King's to change its position or consider removing the damaging statement about the AMP on its website. While the Trust agreed that the CMACE Report was 'not entirely satisfactory', it maintained that the Practice was unsafe for families and unsafe contractually, and stated that there was no intention to carry out an evaluation of King's maternity outcomes. Despite further letters from the NCT and AIMS, there was to be no movement on the Trust's part towards removing the statement on its website. And despite further calls from politicians (including Baroness Cumberlege), academics, health professionals and members of the public, King's would not entertain evaluating its own maternity services.

Communications with the CQC brought no further joy. While the Mums had been unable to get through to anyone who would help them despite 15 emails and endless phone calls, the NCT was immediately able to talk to its Commissioner. It was told that meetings had already taken place between the CQC and King's, and that a plan of action had been put in place following the

CMACE Report. The Commissioner also said she was aware that the NCT and others had called for the removal of the statement on King's website about the AMP being unsafe, but that King's were 'sticking to their guns'. AIMS wrote to the CQC in April 2010 requesting a full review of King's maternity services, but was told that this would not be necessary. A response to Baroness Cumberlege's similar request indicated that the CQC was 'satisfied that the action taken [by King's] was measured and appropriate in minimising any risk to patient safety and quality of treatment.'

AIMS also wrote directly to the CMACE Chair, Professor James Walker, listing concerns about the CMACE Report and including some of the critiques. His short reply absolved CMACE of any responsibility, saying that the review had been correctly carried out and confidentiality maintained. He stated: 'I am fully satisfied that the panels undertook their work independently and objectively'. Tellingly, he also said, as mentioned before: 'the actions subsequently taken by the Trust, which did not include adoption of our recommendations, are a matter for them to explain'.

The campaign's attempts to engage the help of senior politicians met with similar indifference. Letters and briefing papers were sent from the Action Group to the then Secretary of State for Health, Andy Burnham, and to David Cameron, then Leader of the Opposition, in December 2009. Replies came from the Customer Services Centre stating that 'It is the Department of Health's view that King's College Hospital NHS Foundation Trust followed appropriate procedures to protect the safety of patients when deciding to terminate the contract with the Albany Midwifery Practice' and that in any case it was a 'local matter'. A further letter from the NCT to David Cameron, just prior to him being elected Prime Minister, asked him to intervene on behalf of the Albany Midwifery Practice in order to save the model of care for the wellbeing of families. In his response he claimed to be broadly in agreement with the NCT's concerns about the over-medicalisation of childbirth. But the Conservative Party's commitment to privatising healthcare by divesting itself of accountability and leaving this to individual Trusts, meant that he would not intervene in local healthcare arrangements. Ironically, the letter stated:

> 'one of our principles that we support and wish to see extended to the NHS is the freedom of Foundation Trusts to make their own decisions on the basis of the needs and wishes of their local community. For that reason, I don't believe that it would be appropriate for me to pass comment on King's College Hospital's decision on the Albany contract'.

A similar response came from the Department of Health on 28 January 2010, from Anne Keen MP, Under Secretary of State for Health. Again the termination of the Albany contract was deemed to be 'a local matter between the Trust and the midwives and not a matter in which the Department of Health should be involved'. Like the Mums, the Action Group found that powerful institutions were seemingly impenetrable, with no one willing to hold King's to account.

An apparent breakthrough came in early February 2010 when members of the Albany Action Group became aware that they could take their case to the local Health and Adult Services Scrutiny Committee. The Committee had 'a remit to look at the provision of healthcare services and adult social care in the borough'. It was made up of five elected councillors who could 'make reports or recommendations to the council and its health partners'.

King's termination of the Albany contract was added to the Lambeth Scrutiny Committee agenda for 23 February. Members of the campaign were invited to make written submissions and to attend in person with the possibility of making short statements and asking questions. King's was asked to prepare a written report for the agenda, and a representative of the Trust was asked to attend the meeting to answer questions from the committee. Submissions were sent, and members of the Albany Mums, AIMS and NCT attended the meeting, along with the midwives. Facing the Scrutiny Committee were representatives from King's including Roland Sinker (Director of Operations) and Katie Yiannouzis. One of the most striking moments for the campaigners was when one of the councillors wanted to check with the King's managers that she had correctly heard one of their statements – namely that King's claimed to have terminated the contract with the midwives on the grounds of safety, yet was offering all the Albany midwives jobs at King's. Zoe commented afterwards that 'the scrutiny committee people had their jaws on the floor practically. They just couldn't make sense of what they were saying'.

Following the meeting, the campaigners felt that this had been a positive opportunity to discuss their case in public. They felt that the committee had understood why the community felt so aggrieved and that it would be able to take action on the parents' behalf. The committee resolved that King's

> 'should look more closely at its processes in relation to the circumstances around the termination of the contract with the Albany Midwifery Practice and that the issues brought to the debate by the midwives and mothers need to be addressed'.

The committee was also concerned that the breakdown in the relationship between King's and the midwives should not undermine the model of care. The campaigners also took their case to the Scrutiny Committee in the neighbouring borough, where they had another favourable response. Hopes were high that action would follow, but these were dashed. It turned out that while the committees were able to write to King's with recommendations, they had no power to call the Trust to account. King's simply wrote back justifying its actions and explaining why it would not be taking up the committees' recommendations.

Meanwhile, the possibility of both a judicial review* and a

---

* A judicial review is a type of court proceeding in which a judge reviews the lawfulness of a decision or action taken by a public body.

defamation claim against King's were being pursued through legal routes. In the end, after careful consideration of the costs and implications, it was decided not to take either of these further.

One of the main events organised by the Mums and the Action Group was a national march in London on 7 March 2010. The march, held under the banner 'Reclaiming Birth', focused on the Albany model of care and gained national support, including from the RCM, ARM, AIMS, the NCT and Independent Midwives UK.

On a bright, cold day, over 2,000 parents, children, grandparents, midwives, campaigners and many other Albany model supporters, following a double-decker campaign bus, marched with placards, flags, drums, Rix's songs and whistles from Peace Garden at the Imperial War Museum, over Westminster Bridge to Whitehall in London. People came from all over the country demanding more choice for women during childbirth, respect for women's decisions and care from known and trusted midwives. A group of 'Airedale Mums' from Yorkshire, who had long been campaigning for an AMP model

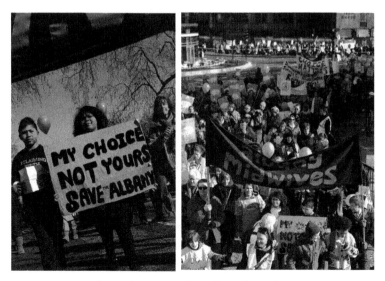

Campaigners marching through London

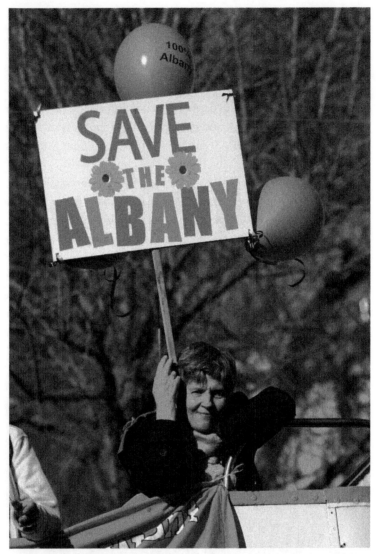

Becky with placard at the Reclaiming Birth rally

in their area, travelled to London by coach to support the call for caseloading midwifery. On arrival at Whitehall, Becky Reed and Emma Beamish, along with speakers from the RCM, AIMS and the NCT, gave speeches from the top of the bus about the value

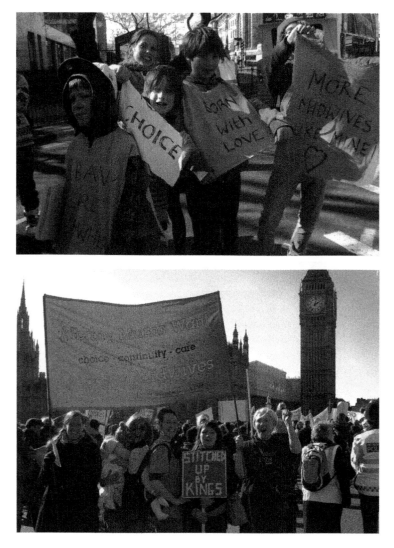

Children and Albany Mums on the march

of the Albany model of midwifery care. Despite wide public support for the march, the campaigners were disappointed that such an important event in the centre of London wasn't covered by either the national press or TV news.

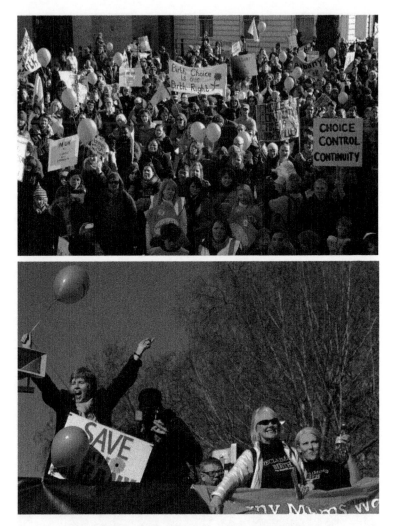

Above: *Campaigners gather in Whitehall.*
Below: *Becky, Pauline and Emma on the campaign bus*

It often felt to the campaigners that all their time, energy and expertise was not achieving results, but their tenacity continued to keep the Albany Midwifery Practice on the King's agenda, as well as in the press and in midwifery and childbirth journals.

The ongoing campaign and the issues it raised inspired Dr Luke

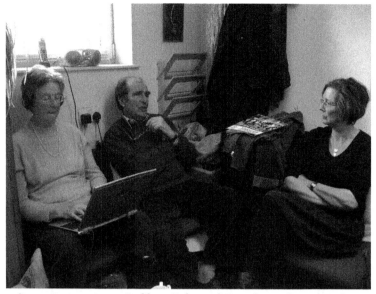

Campaign meeting at Peckham Pulse with Beverley, Luke and Nadine

Zander to set up a remarkable initiative. Luke is a well-respected and influential individual, who practised as a GP for over 30 years in South London. He has a special interest in community-based maternity services, and was a founding member of the Royal Society of Medicine's Maternity and Newborn Forum. Having practised in close proximity to the area where the Albany Midwifery Practice was situated, he was acutely aware of the positive impact that the Practice had had on the outcomes for women and babies in Peckham.

Because of Luke's standing in the maternity world, he had many contacts among midwifery leaders, researchers and activists, some of whom he invited to come to a meeting at the RCM in April 2010, where the Albany Model Advisory Group (AMAG) was formed. The group wanted to better understand the context of the AMP closure in order to campaign for the Albany model of care to be seen as a blueprint for future maternity services, and to address the damaging impact of the closure not only on the AMP, but also on other midwifery continuity schemes. The group was also determined to find a way to compel King's to remove the harmful statement on its website. This had been identified by AMAG as a barrier to advancing the Albany model of midwifery care. The statement was deemed to be inaccurate and defamatory to the midwives and the model, and as long as it remained on King's website it was very difficult to argue for the wider replication of the Albany model of care.

Over a period of more than six years a great many attempts were made by AMAG and others to get King's to remove the statement, but this proved to be very difficult. AMAG arranged a meeting with Tim Smart and Katie Yiannouzis to discuss this and other issues, but the meeting was unsatisfactory and the statement remained on the website. AMAG continued to meet until 2014, and with its support Luke organised a conference in November 2014 at the Royal Society of Medicine in London. The conference, 'Looking back to the future', was held under the auspices of the Maternity and Newborn Forum and focused on relational midwifery care based on the Albany model. Becky gave a keynote presentation, titled 'Lest we forget', on the importance and achievements of the Albany Midwifery Practice.

In the end it was yet another letter from the indefatigable Beverley Beech, Chair of AIMS, to Tim Smart in January 2015 that finally achieved what the campaigners had been requesting for so long. She received the following reply in February, agreeing to remove the damaging statement:

> *Although our position is unchanged regarding our decision in 2009 to terminate the contract with the Albany Midwives practice, we do acknowledge that this statement is no longer relevant to our service and it appears that removal of this statement has been overlooked. As this statement serves no purpose now we are happy to remove it from our website'.*

After six years this felt like a huge achievement.

In the same way that the Albany Mums had felt stonewalled

by King's, the members of the wider campaign met the same resistance. As Pauline remarked, there was no pressure on King's to engage, because there was no mechanism for holding it to account or to compel it to reconsider its decisions.

> 'Once they'd suspended us from practising, they could rest on their laurels, couldn't they? It wasn't an emergency for them any more, so as far as they were concerned they'd stopped this dangerous practice. And all they had to do was sit it out, basically'.

For the wider campaign there still remained two further aims: to clear the names of both Becky and the Albany Practice.

Andy Beckingham FFPH MRSTMH
Consultant in Public Health, Research Fellow, Fernandez Foundation

In 2011, in Hyderabad, India, I had a brief to design a midwifery programme. India didn't have what many Western countries would recognise as midwifery. Maternity care was provided by obstetricians, assisted by a subordinate cadre of 'nurse/midwives' with a nursing ethos. Overloaded obstetricians struggled to cope, and with 26 million births a year, and grossly overloaded public hospitals crammed with impoverished women, 'care' was often dehumanised, neglectful and abusive. In many private hospitals, intervention rates had soared, often unsupported by clinical indication.

By contrast, Fernandez Hospitals aimed to provide high-quality maternal and neonatal care. Dr Evita, an obstetrician who had worked alongside midwives in the NHS, and was now running her own hospitals in Hyderabad, wanted to know whether midwifery could work in India for women with low-risk pregnancies, enabling her obstetricians to focus on care for women at higher risk instead. We began by borrowing midwifery education, curricula and standards from UK universities and the NMC, and the International Confederation of Midwives.

We needed two other things: a woman-centred midwifery philosophy and service model, plus an expert UK midwife to come and demonstrate exemplary midwifery values, behaviour and practice. The Albany Midwifery Practice's remarkable successes, published on its website, showed that it was a 'gold standard' for the rest of the UK to aspire to, particularly for disadvantaged women. We adopted its standards and principles to underpin our programme. And thanks to a misguided, highly persecutory (and later to be dismissed) 'witch hunt' against Becky Reed by the NMC, she happened to be free. We were hugely fortunate to recruit her as our first tutor.

Becky came to Hyderabad to mentor and teach the Indian trainees. They rapidly absorbed midwifery philosophy, theory and practical concepts from her. She began clinical work with them in the labour rooms. Within a fortnight, I was hearing stories of how women in labour had been peering around the curtains where Becky and the trainees were supporting women, and asking if they could have that too.

Fernandez Hospital had always been a 'beacon' of high-quality maternity care for India, open to new ideas, and woman-centred midwifery took off there. Becky's Albany roots and values and her ability to advocate successfully also led to an amazing development with huge potential public health benefits. Finding that mother-baby separation at birth was routine, Becky worked with Dr Evita and the paediatricians to reverse it, promoting skin-to-skin contact and breastfeeding in the first hour. Soon afterwards, these became standard midwifery practice throughout the hospital.

Becky was just the first of a number of UK midwives who came to Fernandez Hospital and influenced the development of professional midwifery, and the Fernandez clinicians have shaped it into an Indian form. But Becky's contribution first grounded it as woman-centred, evidence-based and compassionate, at the same time as promoting positive and physiological birth. I designed the initial curriculum, but my biggest contribution was to get Becky to come and lead a quiet revolution in maternity care.

Eleven years on, more than 15,000 Indian women, from Bollywood stars to women from the Afzal Gunj slums in Hyderabad, have had midwife-led antenatal, intrapartum and post-partum care from professional midwives at Fernandez hospitals. With its original roots in Peckham's Albany Midwifery Practice, this woman-centred model of midwifery has been reincarnated as an Indian profession, now being taken up by a number of other Indian states. Analysis has shown the care is safe, satisfying to women and families, and greatly improves outcomes, including particularly high breastfeeding initiation rates.

From a public health perspective, the closure of the Albany Practice was a disaster. Here we had an evidence-based service model that achieved better clinical outcomes and much higher satisfaction among women than the standard NHS model. It was particularly effective among a highly disadvantaged and ethnically-mixed population Thus, had it not been terminated without good cause, the Albany could have been evaluated as a potential model for addressing the significant and enduring problems of higher maternal mortality and morbidity among the UK's BAME communities. The misguided closure of the Albany also set back wider UK progress on improving maternal health and wellbeing by many years. It also damaged any confidence that local communities had in the ability of NHS senior management to consider their wishes. Evidence from India now shows that the core approach of the Albany, used as a model for midwifery, transforms and greatly improves outcomes. With the closure of the Albany Practice, and the consequent discrediting of its model of care, the UK missed a huge opportunity to improve infant health, maternal health and satisfaction, and lifelong health for both.

19
Vindication

'We must speak truth to power and confront ignorance with facts.'
DaShanne Stokes

In January 2010, feeling desperate about the termination of the Albany's contract with King's and the implications for the Albany model of midwifery care, Becky wrote the following email. She sent it to all the midwifery leaders, researchers and birth activists who had shown an interest in the Albany story, whom she felt might be able and willing to help to clear the name of the Practice.

'Dear supporters of the Albany Practice
PLEA FOR HELP!!!
It's 2010, a bright and hopeful New Year. Last year was shocking and devastating for us, as we saw our beloved Practice vilified and destroyed. As I'm sure most of you know, the Albany Practice, for so long held up as a beacon of hope for the future of NHS midwifery, has had its contract terminated with King's College Hospital Trust, and was closed down just before Christmas. The reasons for the closure are given as patient safety and governance issues, but we feel sure there must be more to it than that [...].

We are totally committed to the Albany model of care, and do not believe that this way of working leads to poorer outcomes. We have statistics from over 10 years which clearly show that this is not the case. We need help to clear our name, which has been and continues to be besmirched by King's (see the statement currently on King's website).

Of course we are midwives first and foremost, and don't necessarily have the skills to manage our campaign in the most effective way possible. This is where you come in! We would like to

*draw on the expertise of all our wonderful supporters, to help us
to move forward in this new year. We are asking you to put your
best thinking caps on to help save this model of midwifery care,
and, we believe, the future of midwifery in this country. We know
that between you you represent all that is great about childbirth
and maternity care – and/or have a vision for maternity policy
– therefore we have great faith that together we can not only save
the Albany, but move midwifery forward for the benefit of mothers,
babies, midwives and families.*

*Please let us know what you think we should do. There will be
many ideas, and they will need coordinating, but we have to start
somewhere. We look forward to hearing from you all.*

With all good wishes for the New Year

Becky (Reed)

and all the members of the Albany Practice'

Responses flooded in, expressing horror at what had happened,
and wanting to offer help and support. Julia Cumberlege called
the situation a 'tragedy', and Cathy Warwick (by now General
Secretary of the RCM) said that the RCM's plan was to 'strongly
support the model and midwifery-led care.'

Important as it was to have so much support, it gradually became
clear that an evaluation of all the outcomes from the AMP would
be the most powerful measure of the safety of the Albany model
of care. The missing piece of the jigsaw was a full analysis of the
Practice outcomes over the entire 12.5 years that it had been open.
As the midwives had always kept full records of their outcomes,
this was still possible. Thus the final work of the campaign was to
try and make sure that this full evaluation was done. As Pauline
said: 'Personally I think we won't get very far with King's until we
have good quality data. With it we will be soaring.'

Nicky Leap, who had been one of the original members of
SELMGP, and who was now an Adjunct Professor of Midwifery at
the University of Technology Sydney (UTS) in Australia, contacted
Caroline Homer in the summer of 2012 to ask if she would be

interested in working on the Albany statistics with a view to publishing an article. Caroline was also a professor of midwifery at UTS, a well-respected researcher in the field of midwifery continuity of care, and had had no previous involvement with the Practice. The clinical outcomes from the first 10 years of the Practice had already been evaluated for the '2000 women study' by Jane Sandall and Becky, for a presentation to the International Congress of Midwives in Glasgow in 2008, so there remained the task of inputting the remaining 2.5 years of statistics. Caroline agreed to take a lead on analysing the data, describing it as a 'really important study'.

Between January 2010 and July 2013 Becky was not surprisingly occupied by her NMC investigation (see Chapter 20), but by autumn 2013 she was ready to organise a 'Where next?' meeting. Campaigners gathered at Becky's house. The group continued to number around 15 committed supporters. In September 2014, still determined to find some answers, Becky wrote to them:

'Dear All

Ok so the holidays are over, it's been more than a year since my NMC hearing, things are obviously moving on for us all...

I've done lots of thinking about where to go next with all the horrible happenings of the last few years, and decided that the biggest priority is the vindication of the Albany Practice Model of Care. Everywhere I go people are talking about what happened, most of them still wide-eyed with disbelief! With the benefit of distance – FIVE YEARS this December since the Practice was closed down – I think it would be a good idea to come together and have a look at what we can do and how we can do it, for those of us who are still fired up enough to give it a go!

So I'm suggesting a meeting with anyone who's interested, and then a campaign to try and get to the bottom of what really happened...

With love to you all, let's VAP*!!!

Becky xx

*Vindicate the Albany Practice'

And thus 'Vindicate the Albany Practice', or 'VAP', became the campaign group's new name. The determination to achieve this vindication showed in the number of people who remained involved, or who joined to support this objective. It was felt that it was important to focus on vindicating the Albany model of care, rather than simply the AMP, so the campaign name was changed to 'VAM' (Vindicate the Albany Model'). Everyone remained keen to 'set the record straight', and all were determined to get the facts out in the open.

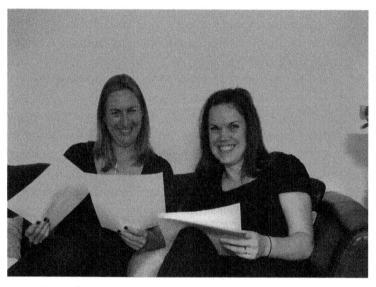

Zoe and Mary working at a campaign meeting, August 2010

While waiting for Caroline Homer's paper to be published the campaign members discussed other ideas to keep the issue of the closure in the public domain. In the end, the final publication of the statistics paper, with its statement: 'Implications for practice: consideration should be given to making similar models of care available to all women' was felt to be enough.

In the lead up to publication, excitement mounted. It could not be overestimated just how important this final analysis could be. In March 2016, Becky enthusiastically wrote to a friend:

'When you think about it, it's pretty amazing how assiduously we kept the data we did keep from the very beginning... but then, we were on a mission of course, to prove that our model of care would work for women and babies.'

In February 2017 the paper was finally accepted for publication in *Midwifery*, a leading international journal in midwifery and maternal health. *Midwifery* is published by Elsevier, whose mission is to 'help researchers and healthcare professionals advance science and improve health outcomes for the benefit of society'. Elsevier states '*Midwifery* publishes the latest peer reviewed international research to inform the safety, quality, outcomes and experiences of pregnancy, birth and maternity care for childbearing women, their babies and families.' The precious Albany statistics were in good hands.

A few days after its acceptance for publication, the paper was published online as an open access article, titled 'Midwifery continuity of care in an area of high socio-economic disadvantage in London: A retrospective analysis of Albany Midwifery Practice outcomes using routine data (1997–2009)'. (The paper is reproduced in part in Appendix I.) This title, while not being the most concise or 'catchy', was designed no doubt to capture the maximum number of people seeking to access information via an internet search engine. It also expresses very well the painstaking work that had been undertaken by the authors of the paper, as they sought to describe the evidence from the full 12.5 years of outcomes from the Albany model of care. The rationale for this work is explained in the paper:

'In light of the unique nature of the Albany Midwifery Practice, its influence on policy, practice and research, its high profile in the international midwifery arena, and the unresolved controversy around the closing of the practice, an independent examination of the maternal and neonatal outcomes over a period of 12 and a half years was seen as critical, hence this evaluation was undertaken.'

When looking at the results of the evaluation, it is of course imperative to understand the context. The AMP had been situated in the borough of Southwark in south-east London, at the time ranked as the 14th most deprived district of 354 districts in England. During the time the Albany Practice was open, Southwark had the highest proportion of babies born with low or very low birth weights; babies of mothers born in East and West Africa and the Caribbean; and babies of mothers who identified as sole parents during the birth registration process.

All women booked with the Albany Midwifery Practice were included in the analysis. As has been described earlier, the midwives provided care for *all* women, regardless of any perceived obstetric, medical or social risk. Of the 2,568 women whose outcomes were analysed, more than half (57%) were from Black, Asian and Minority Ethnic (BAME) communities. (This is the terminology used in the paper, although in 2021 the Commission on Race and Ethnic Disparities recommended that the term BAME be 'disaggregated', in order to better focus on understanding disparities and outcomes for specific ethnic groups.)

Women from BAME groups and single women are both in categories known to be associated with poorer neonatal outcomes. One-third of the women included in the Albany analysis were single, and 11.4% reported being single and unsupported. As the proportion of Albany women from BAME communities was known to be considerably higher than the background rates in the UK, the researchers also undertook an analysis comparing the outcomes for BAME and white women who received care from the Albany midwives.

The full paper can be accessed online. However, it is worth describing some of the relevant results here. Almost all women (95.5%) were cared for in labour by either their primary or secondary midwife. There were high rates of spontaneous onset of labour (80.5%), spontaneous vaginal birth (79.8%), home birth (43.5%), initiation of breastfeeding (91.5%), and breastfeeding at 28 days (74.3% exclusively and another 14.8% mixed feeding). The overall rate of caesarean section was 16%. The preterm birth rate was low (5%). There were 15 perinatal deaths (perinatal mortality rate of 5.78 per 1,000 births), two of which were associated with significant congenital abnormalities. There were no intrapartum (in labour) deaths.

These results are astonishing, especially in the context of an ethnically diverse, all-risk caseload in an area of high deprivation. For comparison, the national home birth rate, which had plummeted in the 1970s, was at this time between 2% and 3%. Caesarean section rates were climbing, and in almost all areas were between 20% and 30%. Breastfeeding rates at 6–8 weeks were well below 50%. Most importantly perhaps, the perinatal mortality rate of the Practice, at 5.78 per 1,000, was approximately half that of Southwark, the London borough in which it was situated (11.4 per 1,000 in 2003–05).

Given the outstanding outcomes, the key conclusion from the research is not surprising:

> 'This analysis has shown that the Albany Midwifery Practice demonstrated positive outcomes for women and babies in socially disadvantaged and BAME groups, including those with complex pregnancies and perceived risk factors.'

The published paper was widely shared in the midwifery world, and AIMS very quickly produced a press release, titled 'VINDICATED AT LAST'. The AIMS statement finished with these words:

> 'The Albany Midwifery Practice provided care in exactly the way successive Government policy has strongly recommended since 2003. The research which has just been published lends even more weight to the huge benefits of this model of care – consistently more health and social benefits and less damage to women and babies, no matter what their circumstances.'

Needless to say, the vindication provided by the paper was felt most keenly among those who had worked so hard to show that the Albany model of care truly worked. Becky summed up her feelings in a 'thank you' email to Caroline Homer, the lead author:

> '*Thank you so much for the paper. It will have far-reaching consequences. Today my emotions are all over the place – excited to see it of course, but also very angry (I'm sure you understand why). So much damage caused by King's distortion of the statistics, so much pain and misery to so many. So thank you again for getting the truth out there.*'

Albany midwives' reactions to reading Closure

'Such a compelling read. It is beautifully and eloquently written with hard-hitting evidence of how badly we were treated, and the detrimental effect this had on women, midwives and the future of maternity services.' Danielle

'I have really "enjoyed" reading the book, however it has brought back a lot of anger and sadness about the whole situation. I feel incredulous that it was all allowed to play out as it did.' Nicky

'It was so hard reading it all again as I have blocked a lot of the feelings I had when we were living and working during the investigation process as it was such an awful time. It was such a huge loss for the women we looked after and it was such a loss for us as midwives. The consequences of what they did for me personally were profound…' Fran

'So emotional reading it… It's such a weird mixture of being so excited to read the next bit and can't wait but simultaneously feeling overwhelmed by it, it's quite traumatic. It's such a big thing to finally read this story. It feels important not just for justice and for healing, but for the future.' Natalie

'When you read it, it becomes all the more unbelievable that it ever happened…' Sophie

'This is a much-needed book to tell our story. I still can't quite believe this happened to us, and still feel incredibly sad that the Practice has gone, for women and the greater midwifery world.' Mary

'[You have managed to] get the complex story of the Practice and closure into words on a page. I'm finding it horrific… shocking… desperately sad. I still feel shocked all these years on about the poor quality of the data that all the later events were based on.' Zoe V

'Such an important book for all. It was a very emotional read thinking about my own personal loss… and for the other midwives and the women who lost this exceptional model of midwifery care. And it made me angry, so very angry. How dare they! And they did and they got away with it.' Zoe L

Becky's story: chronology of a witch hunt

additional author Sarah Davies

> *'The suspension (from duty) of one of the Albany Midwives and cessation of her practice reminds me of my own suspension in 1985 [...] the same technique of selecting cases with adverse outcomes without looking at the overall care, and the same refusal to look at what the women themselves want.'* Wendy Savage

This book would not be complete without the story of the investigations into Becky's practice, both by supervisors of midwives at King's College Hospital and by the Nursing and Midwifery Council (NMC). This was a protracted story of institutional failures that ended with no acknowledgement, no apology and no recompense for the significant reputational, financial and emotional damage that these institutions inflicted on Becky and her family over nearly five years.

It all began with supervision. Statutory supervision of midwives came into effect in the UK in the early 20th century, and was designed both to provide support for midwives and protection for the public, by actively promoting a safe standard of midwifery practice. Prior to the Albany closure supervision at King's had been described by senior midwifery managers as 'not working terribly well' and as 'dysfunctional'. In the Department of Health and Social Care Policy Paper of 2016, statutory supervision of midwives was 'criticised, closely examined and found to be flawed', and was changed at government level in 2017.

Investigations into Becky's midwifery practice began in October

2008, when the first supervisory investigation by King's was initiated by Linda Sherratt (Risk Management Midwife) following the birth of a baby born in unexpectedly poor condition (Case 1). Becky was the second midwife in attendance at this birth. Although aware that the investigation should be happening, and indeed should be completed within 20 days, Becky heard nothing for several months. She finally received a request to attend a supervisory interview on 25 February 2009. In a phone call the investigating supervisor said that she had been asked to look at six extra cases where Becky had been one of the midwives. Becky was aware that widening an investigation in this way contravened the guidelines for supervisory practice. She emailed the supervisor asking for clarification but received no reply.

Becky attended the interview, supported by her personal supervisor Kate Brintworth. Knowing the guidelines, Kate started by asking for confirmation that this interview was solely to do with Case 1. The supervisor seemed confused, but eventually admitted that she had been given seven cases for 'overall review', in order to look for 'underlying similarities in these cases'. Aware that this now seemed more and more like a 'fishing expedition', rather than an investigation into a single case, Becky felt she had no option but to request that the meeting be ended. Although this meeting was supposed to be confidential under the rules of supervision, Consultant Obstetrician Leonie Penna commented to an Albany midwife in the corridor just minutes later that she had heard that Becky was 'not cooperating' with the investigation.

Consultant midwife Cathy Walton, who was already concerned about the standard of midwifery supervision at King's, was so worried about what had happened that she immediately wrote a letter of complaint to Angela Helleur, the Local Supervising Authority Midwifery Officer (LSAMO). Following this, the handling of Becky's investigation was taken over by the Deputy LSAMO, and out of the hands of King's. This investigation was concluded on 18 March 2009, and resulted in Becky being required to undertake 'supported practice' in order to continue working as a midwife. And yet, two days prior to this decision the inquest into the baby's death had found that there had been *no evidence of neglect on the part of the midwives*. In finding Becky culpable and imposing such a sanction were the supervisors unaware of this finding, or had they simply chosen to ignore it?

In July 2009 another investigation was begun into Becky's practice (Case 2). This time the supervisory report focused mainly on the issue of blood sugar monitoring for a borderline low birth weight baby. Although this monitoring was recommended in King's guidelines, the mother had made an informed decision to decline. It was suggested that Becky had failed to communicate to her the risks of low blood sugar in a newborn baby, but this had in fact been discussed in detail. Ironically, while carrying out a lengthy period of supervised practice based on this case at Barnet and Chase Farm Hospital in London, Becky discovered that the guidelines there were different from those at King's. Had the baby been born at Barnet and Chase Farm, he would not have been considered to be at risk, and his blood sugar would not have been routinely monitored.

During the supervisory investigation into Case 2, on 28 September 2009, Becky attended a planned home birth (Case 3). The baby was born in good condition but collapsed 25 minutes after birth, and died several days later. At the long-delayed inquest into the baby's death, there was again a finding of 'no evidence of neglect'. (The full story of this birth is covered in detail in Chapter 13.) Following this tragic event, with King's lacking awareness of the facts and disbelieving the midwives' accounts of what had happened, Becky was suspended from duty with no offer of support. And thus began a third supervisory hearing.

By now the supervisory reports into Cases 1 and 2 had wrongly accused Becky of numerous examples of poor practice. In October she submitted a detailed complaint to the LSA about both the process and the content of the first of the two supervisory investigations. She was then dismayed to discover that there was no mechanism for challenging inaccurate content in a supervisory investigation report; it was only possible to challenge the process.

The questioning of Becky's practice was unrelenting. In January 2010, a month after the decision to close the Albany Practice, she was referred to the NMC by Katie Yiannouzis, Head of Midwifery at King's and Becky's former supervisor of midwives. The referral focused primarily on Case 3, but also included the six other cases mentioned above. Becky later reflected:

> 'I think what happened was… they went fishing, and looked for any case that had been risk managed where I'd been involved to add to their list of allegations. So even though there hadn't been any negligence… they still saw fit to use them as part of their wider referral'.

Katie's referral to the NMC broke a number of rules. She failed to tell Becky that she had referred her, and she also failed to inform the LSA, although on the form she stated that this had been done. Becky only found out about the referral second-hand a few weeks later, after discovering that Katie had written letters to several women, asking for permission to disclose a copy of their medical records to the NMC. In the letters to the women Katie explained that due to concerns about some of Becky's care she had 'taken the serious step' of reporting her to the Nursing and Midwifery Council. This had unsurprisingly caused the women distress and confusion.

Feeling in need of support, Becky phoned Cathy Warwick, now Chief Executive of the RCM. Cathy expressed her concern and astonishment that 'King's was digging [these cases] up'. She advised Becky to contact Francine Allen, RCM Regional Officer, as soon as possible. On hearing the story, Francine declared herself to be 'pole-axed', and set about trying to find out from the NMC whether there had indeed been a referral.

Meanwhile, Becky wrote to Katie asking her to confirm the referral, but received no response. At the end of March she wrote to Tim Smart, King's CEO:

'I have heard nothing from the NMC to say that I have been reported to them. I have spoken to the LSA Midwifery Officer, who would normally be kept informed in such a situation, and she was unaware of any referral. I wrote to Katie on the 9th March, asking for an explanation; as I have had no reply (nor even an acknowledgment) from her, I feel that I now need to make you aware of her actions. I wrote to her again yesterday, and I am attaching a copy of that letter for your information...'

Tim Smart replied immediately saying 'your email has raised some important issues', and that he would reply after a short investigation. However, in spite of continuing requests for information, and with no satisfactory response forthcoming, Becky was becoming increasingly frustrated and upset. It wasn't until the very end of April, three months after she had initially heard rumours about her referral, that Katie finally confirmed to Becky that she had indeed referred her to the NMC. In her letter, Katie described herself as the 'nominated person' to do this, as Chair of the Risk Management Committee. It seemed extraordinary that a Head of Midwifery, who had in the past been Becky's supervisor, and had even offered her a midwifery post at King's, had at the same time referred her to the regulatory body for apparent misconduct.

Becky continued to press both Tim Smart and Katie Yiannouzis for the details of her referral, and Tim Smart finally sent her a copy of the referral letter on 22 June. In his email he made the following comment, unilaterally closing down communication:

'I will not enter into any further correspondence with you regarding this matter and I ask that you refrain from further contacting Mrs Yiannouzis or any other King's staff about it.'

When Becky's NMC referral became public, midwives, academics and activists across the UK and internationally were appalled by the vexatious and incompetent investigations to which she was being subjected. They recognised that she was being scapegoated. Four of them, Sarah Davies, Nadine Edwards, Mavis Kirkham and Jo Murphy-Lawless (Becky later referred to them as her 'Fearsome Foursome'), sent a letter to the LSAMO, Angela Helleur, in May 2010, signed by 117 senior midwives and activists. The letter criticised the supervisory investigations and called for Becky's suspension to be revoked. In spite of this the supervisory and NMC investigations continued.

Becky finally received the NMC 'Notice of Referral' in July 2010, along with the first 'bundle' of documentation. Her husband Adrian recalls her saying:

> 'They've picked the wrong person. If I was a young midwife, this would destroy me. I now have nothing to lose – and I'll fight this all the way.'

The 'bundle' contained documents relating to seven cases of women and babies where Becky had been involved, going back to 2006. Becky had been primary midwife in only three of these cases; the primary midwives had not been referred. The allegations made against her were so general that it was impossible for her to respond: allegations such as 'Failed to meet the required standard of a competent Midwife' and 'Drafted documentation which was inaccurate or contradictory'.

In early September 2010 Becky was notified that an Interim Order hearing at the NMC would be held two weeks later to decide whether or not she should be allowed to continue practising. Becky was unable to attend for family reasons, and requested that the hearing be delayed. The RCM representative, Pat Gould, told her this would not be possible and reassured her that she would be well represented. In the event, Pat was extremely ill-prepared, muddling her papers and failing to explain to the panel the circumstances of the referral or to describe Becky's exemplary practice. After considering the allegations, and with Becky not able to be present to argue her case, the NMC panel ruled that she must undertake 450 hours (the maximum possible) of supervised practice if she wanted to remain on the register.

After the panel ruling Becky said in a letter to a friend:

> 'I'm trying to keep focused on why I'm going through all this. At my age I could have just caved in, stopped practising, retired, played with my grandchildren. But this is a fight that has to be fought for midwives (and women and babies) in the future'.

Unfortunately the RCM, the professional body that should have supported Becky in her fight, continued to be weak and ineffective throughout the NMC investigation. Sarah Davies, senior lecturer in midwifery at Salford University, wrote to the RCM questioning 'its muted and tentative response... which has ramifications for the confidence of midwives across the UK as they attempt against the odds to lead woman centred care in line with government policy... I am mystified as to why the RCM isn't backing Becky as publicly as possible'.

Becky then spent the winter of 2010–2011 completing the 450 hours of supervised practice at Barnet and Chase Farm hospitals, many miles from her home. Some of the midwives at Chase Farm knew of Becky from her published articles in a midwifery journal, *The Practising Midwife*, and were surprised to see her there on supervised practice. Becky was in an extraordinary position at this time: looked up to by midwives and students alike, and at the same time told that she was not allowed to be on her own with either a woman or a baby. On one occasion she attended an update study day on breech birth, only to find photographs from one of her own cases being used to illustrate best practice.

Becky was signed off from her supervised practice with glowing references in April 2011. Following this, a second NMC Interim Order Review was held on 21 April. Eighty heartfelt testimonials from parents and midwives had been submitted to the Fitness to Practice panel. Pat Gould, the RCM representative, declared herself to be unhappy about this, saying that they should be 'proper professional testimonials on headed notepaper, rather than [from] acquaintances and women [she] had cared for in the past'.

At the hearing, however, the panel was impressed by the testimonials. Each one was a powerful and moving personal story describing the life-changing effects of Becky's midwifery care on individual mothers, families, midwives and student midwives. One of the mothers, Angela, said:

> 'Becky was my main midwife with my first child. She was with me during my pregnancy and reassuring me all the way before and after the birth. At all times Becky encouraged me and my partner. When she monitored my labour she made sure that all this information was written to a great detail.
>
> With my second child, as soon as she found out that I was in labour she turned up to help me. Again after the birth of my daughter, she helped me to get the basics right and to look after my baby. She made me believe in myself when I didn't. She showed me how to deliver safely my daughter and to look after my son after a caesarean.
>
> Becky is not only a midwife, she is a networker as well. She has looked after people of all backgrounds, and does not leave anybody out. I pray that she is allowed to carry on doing the amazing job that she has done for so many years and that this situation ends.'

Based on her references and the testimonials, the NMC Fitness to Practice panel ruled that Becky was fit to practise without restrictions. However the NMC's Investigating Committee then made the incomprehensible decision to continue its case against Becky. As barrister Elizabeth Prochaska commented:

> 'It was this faceless bureaucracy that just had no time really to consider what it was doing... And there seemed to be no way to stop it, no way to just say, "Hello, look at what's really going on?"'

Elizabeth Prochaska was a human rights barrister who was also working at the time as a doula. She had heard the story of the

Albany Practice, had offered her expertise, and went on to support Becky during the remaining 15 months of her investigation.

Becky was by now becoming used to 'bundles' of paperwork arriving from the NMC. In April 2011, the same month that she was declared fit to practise, she received yet another 'bundle'. However, the NMC this time had made a monumental error, enclosing 30 pages of confidential information relating to a different midwife's NMC case. Ironically, with the papers came a warning: 'if you do not take proper steps to protect confidential information, this may result in another allegation regarding your fitness to practise'. Found to be guilty themselves, the NMC did manage to apologise for this serious breach of confidentiality. It turned out to be the only apology Becky ever received.

Despite the huge pressure of the investigation, Becky still continued to make a difference to the lives of women and babies. In summer 2011 she was invited to work as a midwifery consultant to an innovative training programme for midwives in Hyderabad in India which was being designed by Andy Beckingham, a public health consultant from the UK. He had identified the Albany Practice as a model of care that could be adapted for the needs of Indian women. Because of the continuing NMC investigation Becky was available, and between September 2011 and July 2012 she visited Fernandez Hospitals in Hyderabad, mentoring and teaching the first group of professional midwifery students in India, and working with them to implement evidence-based practice. Andy had based the programme on the Albany Practice's woman-centred philosophy and service model, and later said: 'We were hugely fortunate to recruit [Becky] as our first tutor... without her contribution, it would have been extremely difficult to bring about such a high level of clinical outcome improvement.'

In March 2012, at home in London between her visits to Hyderabad, Becky received yet another bundle, this time with the results of the NMC investigation. She was shocked to see 63 draft charges against her, based on five of the original seven cases, with a demand for a response to these charges within 28 days. But the papers in the bundle only contained the notes for one of the cases, making it difficult to properly respond. Becky therefore requested the notes for the other four cases (one of which dated back nearly six years) but was told less than a week before her response was due that the notes were 'not disclosable'.

The main part of this bundle was the NMC's expert witness report by Beverley Lynn, a midwife with no obvious relevant credentials and no track record of performing such a role. She had relied heavily on the discredited CMACE Report provided by the NMC, which, given that it was about the Practice as a whole and not about Becky personally, was not relevant to the investigation. However, the NMC had failed to supply Beverley with material which *was* relevant, such as the findings of the two inquests into cases 1 and 3, the risk management reports from King's, the result of the previous NMC investigation into Case 1 which had found 'no case to answer', and the report of Becky's supervised practice. Needless to say, Beverley Lynn's report was full of mistakes. As Elizabeth Prochaska remarked:

> 'The expert report itself, when it arrived, was riddled with errors. For example, it said one of the babies died, when it didn't, which is a pretty fundamental error. (...) The expert report seemed to rely on sources that frankly had nothing to do with Becky's practice – the CMACE Report. The report talked about the practice of other midwives when that wasn't relevant to what it was meant to be doing. I mean, it was very poor'.

Despite not having the midwifery case notes for four of the five cases, Becky drew on her own documentation. With help from Elizabeth Prochaska she put together the following response to the draft charges, which was sent to the NMC on 25 April 2012:

Case 1
I was the second midwife in this case, and arrived late in the labour to support the primary midwife. Following a risk management

investigation I was required to complete a Programme of Developmental Support. This was signed off successfully on 21 July 2009. The parents referred both midwives to the NMC. After I had responded to the allegations, the Investigating Committee decided that there was no case to answer. In my opinion the Investigating Committee should be very slow to reverse the findings of a previous committee without fresh and compelling new evidence. I have not been advised of any such evidence.

Case 2 (baby did not die as stated in the draft charges)
Please note that the charges in this case have been drafted without access to the patient records. I was the primary midwife in this case, although due to her prolonged pregnancy I was on holiday at the time the baby was admitted to hospital post-delivery. A supervisory investigation into this incident was so badly completed that I challenged the process, although LSA rules did not allow me to challenge the content. My challenge was upheld overall and the supervisor was directed to 'review her report'. In the event the recommendation arising out of the flawed report (that I complete a maximum period of supervised practice) was upheld. My supervised practice imposed at the Interim Orders Hearing related to this case. As stated above, this was completed and signed off on 5 April 2011, following which at the Interim Order Review Hearing my conditions of practice were entirely revoked.

Case 3
I was the primary midwife in this case, which was an uncomplicated home birth of a third baby. The baby collapsed with a cardio-respiratory arrest 25 minutes after delivery. The inquest into the death of this baby found no evidence of neglect on the part of the midwives. The Expert Witness [at the inquest] found that the baby had had a period of antepartum hypoxia, which we could not have identified. The Coroner concluded that the 'death was due to the effects of chronic hypoxia commencing about two days prior to delivery followed by cardio-respiratory arrest shortly after delivery'.

Case 4

This was a historic case, dating back almost six years. I was the second midwife in this case, and arrived half way through the labour to act in a supporting role. At no point did I 'take over care' as stated in the draft charge. The risk management report on this incident (...) stated 'The midwives conducted the breech delivery appropriately...' The risk management report also states 'The midwives and medical staff appear to have had good communication during delivery allowing the doctor to attend rapidly when required.' The allegation that I did not obtain timely medical assistance is therefore unjustified. It is worth noting that [the mother] requested that I attend her for the birth of her next child in 2008.

Case 5

This case dates back over four years. I was the second midwife in this case, called in to help by the first midwife and never having met the woman before. I arrived when she was in advanced labour with an undiagnosed breech. The woman had chosen a Caesarean section, but there was an emergency in theatre and the obstetricians failed to open a second theatre. When the woman finally got to theatre, she was fully dilated and the breech was descending. A decision was made by the doctors to attempt a vaginal delivery. The labour ward was full with no rooms available; we were told to stay in theatre for the birth, a highly unsatisfactory situation. The birth occurred reasonably quickly and we were left alone by the doctors to look after the woman. We had some concerns about the CTG [a device for monitoring the baby's wellbeing] *but were reassured by the doctors. We called a paediatrician to attend the birth; the doctors arrived at the last minute. The risk management report in this case focused mainly on organisational and staff issues. There was no supervisory investigation and no midwifery sanctions at the time.*

At the same time as Becky was preparing her response to the NMC, the *British Journal of Midwifery* (BJM) was inviting nominations for its Practice Awards, to 'celebrate the fantastic work that UK midwives perform in today's challenging healthcare environment'. The *BJM* was deluged with emails nominating Becky for the Lifetime Achievement Award. She was shortlisted and invited to the gala dinner, and her chosen guest had even bought her train ticket from Manchester, but at the very last minute the *BJM* informed her that their rules precluded giving an award to any midwife under investigation.

The investigation continued for several more months, until in early autumn 2012 Becky was suddenly informed that the NMC had decided to change its remit. It was no longer looking at her historical practice, but was now focusing on her *current* fitness to practise. Did this mean that the 63 charges, still publicly accessible on the NMC website, were no longer relevant?

Based on this extraordinary development, Pat Gould recommended that Becky get a midwifery job in which she could prove herself to be a safe practitioner. Jackie Moulla, now Becky's supervisor, was working as a Consultant Midwife at Whipps Cross Hospital in London, and suggested applying for a vacancy at the Birth Centre there. Becky mustered all her strength to prepare herself for an interview. In spite of needing to declare her current status as a midwife under investigation, she got the job and prepared to go back into clinical practice. She wrote to Pat Gould:

> 'I just wanted to let you know that I have been offered a job as a Band 6 midwife, on the Birth Centre at Whipps Cross Hospital. My work in India is on hold for the moment, and I am concentrating on maximising my chances of getting through my NMC case with the best possible outcome. I just really hope it helps when the time comes for my hearing. Needless to say I am looking forward to getting back to some clinical midwifery, and working with women and babies again.'

However, the job on the Birth Centre didn't last long. Within a week the managers got cold feet about Becky's status as a midwife under investigation, and insisted on moving her to the high-risk labour ward, where she then worked for six months in an unfamiliar and often hostile environment. The strategy of taking the job paid off, however, and she was eventually able to present some very favourable testimonials to the final hearing panel in July the following year.

Meanwhile the campaign to support Becky, and the midwifery knowledge, skills and philosophy that she represented, continued to gather momentum. Inspired by the campaign, activist Vicky Garner volunteered to set up a Facebook page Justice for Midwife Becky Reed (JFMBR) in January 2013. The page soon had over 2,500 supporters, an impressive number at that time.

The following month Jenny Fraser, Becky's expert witness, completed her report for the NMC. Jenny was a highly respected expert witness and mentor, with 20 years experience in the field. In her report she concluded:

> 'What comes through to me is a genuine commitment to give woman-centred flexible care, which is something we should all strive for. I have not found any actions/omissions, as set out in the draft charges, which make me think in any way that Ms Reed's fitness to practice is impaired.'

Jenny Fraser was due to give evidence at the final two-week hearing of Becky's case, which was planned for March 2013, over three years since she had first been referred. Vicky Garner began to coordinate support for Becky for each day of the two-week hearing. However, only two weeks before the planned date, the NMC postponed the hearing, saying that it had been unable to put together a panel. Soo Downe, a professor of midwifery, wrote on the Facebook page:

> 'I find it incredible that Becky's case has been postponed, at a time when the NMC is so closely under scrutiny, and when it is well

known how important and crucial this case is – quite apart from the appalling lack of concern for Becky's health and wellbeing, and the financial consequences, after all this time'.

The postponed hearing, now inexplicably extended to three weeks, was booked for 15 July to 2 August 2013. Again Becky's supporters rallied, many writing to the NMC CEO Jackie Smith to express their outrage at the way Becky was being treated.

However, in a completely unforeseen move, on 14 June Becky's solicitor informed her that a decision had been made to 'dispose of' her case in a one-day hearing:

'You will see that the NMC have decided that they have no evidence to offer that your fitness to practice is impaired. Effectively they are throwing in the towel'.

This U-turn was both a relief and a blow to Becky. She was relieved at the NMC's decision to offer no evidence, but felt robbed of her opportunity to answer the charges and defend herself publicly. In an email to a friend the following day she wrote:

'Unbelievable… such a huge mixture of emotions, but mainly anger at how I've been treated for nearly 3 and a half years, anger at their stupidity and incompetence, and determination to REALLY get justice at the end and not have it all just swept under a carpet.'

There was an immediate announcement to this effect on the Facebook page:

'JFMBR has very mixed feelings about this. A short one-day hearing will not address the multitude of issues raised, let alone the 63 charges that Becky has been facing and which are now apparently being abandoned. This whole sorry process, which has lasted three and a half years and which has been so damaging to Becky and

her family, has also of course raised issues of great concern for the wider midwifery world.'

As Elizabeth Prochaska commented, the case should never have reached the point it did:

> *'There was no prospect that, even if the case had been heard in full, the NMC was going to get any sanctions. It was just a complete waste of time and money to have a hearing. They should have realised that so much sooner. It was just persecutory. It felt really negligent on their part'.*

In the event, the hearing on 15 July was a travesty of justice. In order to save face, the NMC lawyer suggested that it was only because of the extensive 'remedial' action that Becky had taken, as well as her recent work on a hospital labour ward, that she was now fit to practise: a decision that the NMC Interim Order panel had reached over two years earlier. At the hearing Becky had no opportunity to respond, and the case was dismissed.

> *'Because of the NMC lawyer's decision to offer no evidence in my case, and to dispose of the case at a one-day hearing, the allegations were never addressed. Most of these allegations I did not accept, and almost all of them were dismissed by my expert witness. Because of the NMC lawyer's decision to offer no evidence in my case, I had no opportunity to defend myself.'*

The 63 allegations remained in the public domain on the NMC website for several days following the hearing. The verdict of 'no case to answer' was not reported on the website, and all reference to the case was removed within a few days. It was almost as if the whole thing had never happened.

Unable to attend the hearing due to lack of space, Albany families, campaigners and midwives from all around the country gathered on the day in Lincoln's Inn Fields, not far from the NMC

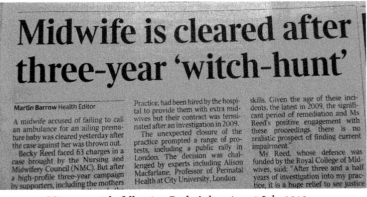

Midwife is cleared after three-year 'witch-hunt'

Martin Barrow Health Editor

A midwife accused of failing to call an ambulance for an ailing premature baby was cleared yesterday after the case against her was thrown out.

Becky Reed faced 63 charges in a case brought by the Nursing and Midwifery Council (NMC). But after a high-profile three-year campaign by supporters, including the mothers

Practice, had been hired by the hospital to provide them with extra midwives but their contract was terminated after an investigation in 2009.

The unexpected closure of the practice prompted a range of protests, including a public rally in London. The decision was challenged by experts including Alison Macfarlane, Professor of Perinatal Health at City University, London.

skills. Given the age of these incidents, the latest in 2009, the significant period of remediation and Ms Reed's positive engagement with these proceedings, there is no realistic prospect of finding current impairment."

Ms Reed, whose defence was funded by the Royal College of Midwives, said: "After three and a half years of investigation into my practice, it is a huge relief to see justice

Times article following Becky's hearing, 3 July 2013

building in London. When the news came through that the hearing had ended, the supporters marched to the NMC building, waving banners and singing campaigning songs written by Rix Pyke. They gathered at the entrance, singing to the theme tune of the TV series *Robin Hood*: 'NMC, NMC this is not the end, NMC, NMC we'll drive you round the bend/ here we will wait, till you exonerate/ Becky Reed, Becky Reed, Becky Reed.'

Becky emerged, flanked by bemused-looking NMC officials, who must never before have witnessed such an occasion. She then spoke movingly about the support she had received from her family, friends and activists, and talked about those midwives who were continuing to face unfair sanctions in the UK and internationally. As Becky embraced her supporters individually, they sang (to the Beatles' tune *Let it be*):

> '*Becky Reed's a midwife full of wisdom and integrity/There is no case to answer NMC/If Becky is the iceberg there are hundreds more beneath the sea/Midwives won't be bullied, Let us be/ NMC, NMC, NMC, NMC Midwives won't be bullied, let us be…*' (See Appendix II for Rix Pyke's full lyrics.)

Vicky Garner commented:

> 'As her family, friends and supporters cheered and sang for her, it was… not just for Becky, but for the beautiful, loving and highly skilled midwifery care that midwife Becky Reed exemplified'.

Becky's supporters, who had devoted vast amounts of time and energy to writing letters and emails, and attending meetings, were outraged that the NMC had taken no responsibility for the damage it had inflicted on Becky, her family and midwifery as a whole. Elizabeth Prochaska commented: 'it was like [Becky] was engaging with a completely faceless monster, you know, who just was never going to recognise her humanity and what this process was doing to her life and to her family's life'.

Unbelievably, from 2008 onwards this 'faceless monster' had been designated a failing organisation by its own regulator, the Council for Healthcare Regulatory Excellence (CHRE). In 2012, even while the NMC was investigating Becky, the CHRE had concluded:

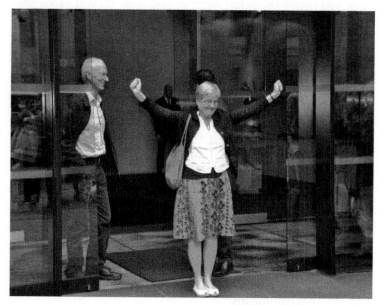

Becky after the hearing with her husband Adrian

'At the heart of the NMC's failure to succeed lies confusion over its regulatory purpose, lack of clear, consistent strategic direction, unbalanced working relationships and inadequate business systems (...) weaknesses in governance, leadership, decision making and operational management'.

Becky's complaint to Jackie Smith, chief executive of the NMC, echoed these damning findings:

'During my investigation the NMC was found by its own regulatory body, the CHRE, to be failing 'at every level' (...) In contrast, I believe I have always acted in an honest, skilled and professional manner; this is reinforced by the findings of the Interim Order panel and the eventual verdict of no case to answer. Yet while I have been treated punitively throughout, as well as required to reflect and show insight, my regulatory body has failed to apply this approach to its own conduct. For three and a half years I experienced a consistently adversarial attitude, inordinate delays, misunderstandings of midwifery and failures of process. I believe that all the above failings amount to misconduct of my regulatory body'.

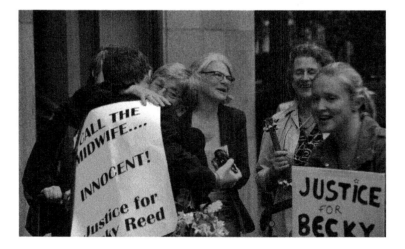

Becky embracing her supporters, with Sarah Davies, Rix Pyke and Becky's daughter Martha

Becky also requested an apology from the NMC and assurances that this destructive process could never happen to another midwife:

> *'I am determined that other midwives should not suffer in the way that I have'.*

She summed up the devastating impact of this catalogue of institutional failings:

> *'The length of the investigation, the restrictions on my practice, and the constant fear and uncertainty, all combined to cause me and my family extreme distress. The impact on my life has been profound, not only from an emotional perspective, but also both professionally and financially'.*

The NMC has never apologised to Becky for the damage it did.

Elizabeth Prochaska
Barrister

We all need good midwifery regulation. Not only to protect the public from poor practice, but because regulation establishes midwives' legitimacy as professionals and enables them to practice within the healthcare system. In countries without midwifery regulation, women often turn to midwives working outside the system, who may then put themselves at risk of prosecution and prison by providing care. The UK's system of midwifery regulation by the Nursing and Midwifery Council (NMC) is often admired in those countries and held up as a system to which they should aspire.

By the time I met Becky in 2011, I had been representing midwives at the NMC for a few years. With each case that I did, my conviction in the NMC's inadequacy became stronger. I saw not only incompetence – lost files, endless delays, inexpert 'experts' – but also an entrenched hostility towards any midwife working outside the mainstream. The NMC regarded these midwives as renegades, regardless of their seniority in the profession or the depth of their knowledge and skills. It accepted hospital standards of care as the only legitimate standards, no matter whether they were evidence-based or met NICE guidelines, and it questioned women's informed decisions to decline those standards, suggesting that they must have been hoodwinked by their midwives. This was a culture clash, and one in which the NMC held the power to destroy reputations and end careers.

When I first met Becky, she was scared and bewildered to find herself under investigation, but she also spoke with a fierce certainty and pride about the Albany. She knew without doubt that the Albany midwives had provided exemplary care. When she brought me her papers, I was ready to believe she could have made a mistake, that there might be something in all those cases that could be criticised. There was not. The NMC's 'allegations' were absurd, a litany of tiny criticisms of Becky's practice, many of them based on factual errors by the NMC, that added up to nothing. But the process ground on; no one in the NMC getting a grip; all oblivious to Becky's suffering. When, after years of unjustified and heartless bureaucratic meandering, the NMC finally engaged properly with the case against her, it disintegrated like ash in their hands. The NMC's case against Becky was a mockery of good regulation that protected no one.

In February 2014, some months after the case against Becky was dismissed, she was my midwife at the birth of my second child. For Becky, I believe this felt like a vindication. I had seen every possible criticism of her, and I chose her as my midwife. For me, it was the only choice. I knew I could not feel safer or be more loved.

Appendix I

Extract from: *Midwifery continuity of care in an area of high socio-economic disadvantage in London: A retrospective analysis of Albany Midwifery Practice outcomes using routine data* (1997–2009)*

Abstract

Objective: in 1997, The Albany Midwifery Practice was established within King's College Hospital NHS Trust in a South East London area of high social disadvantage. The Albany midwives provided continuity of care to around 216 women per year, including those with obstetric, medical or social risk factors. In 2009, the Albany Midwifery Practice was closed in response to concerns about safety, amidst much publicity and controversy. The aim of this evaluation was to examine trends and outcomes for all mothers and babies who received care from the practice from 1997–2009.

Design: a retrospective, descriptive analysis of data routinely collected over the 12.5 year period was undertaken including changes over time and outcomes by demographic features.

Setting and participants: all women booked with the Albany Midwifery Practice were included.

Findings: of the 2568 women included over the 12.5 year period, more than half (57%) were from Black, Asian and Minority Ethnic (BAME) communities; one third were single and 11.4% reported being single and unsupported. Almost all women (95.5%) were cared for in labour by either their primary or secondary midwife. There were high rates of spontaneous onset of labour (80.5%), spontaneous vaginal birth (79.8%), homebirth (43.5%), initiation of breastfeeding (91.5%) and breastfeeding at 28 days (74.3% exclusively and 14.8% mixed feeding). Of the 79% of women who had a physiological third stage, 5.9% had a postpartum haemorrhage. The overall rate of caesarean section was 16%. The preterm birth rate was low (5%). Ninety-five per cent of babies had an Apgar score of 8 or greater at 5 minutes and 6% were admitted to a neonatal unit for more than two days. There were 15 perinatal deaths (perinatal mortality rate of 5.78 per 1000 births); two were associated with significant congenital abnormalities. There were no intrapartum intrauterine deaths.

Key conclusions: this analysis has shown that the Albany Midwifery Practice demonstrated positive outcomes for women and babies in socially disadvantaged and BAME groups, including those with complex

---

* The full text is available at https://www.sciencedirect.com/science/article/pii/S0266613817301511?via%3Dihub

pregnancies and perceived risk factors.

Implications for practice: consideration should be given to making similar models of care available to all women.

Discussion

We undertook this retrospective audit to examine the trends and outcomes for all mothers and babies who received care from the Albany Midwifery Practice during 12 and a half years, from 1997–2009. The Albany Midwifery Practice is a model that was emulated and used as a template for other midwife-led services around the world before the contract was terminated in 2009 due to safety concerns (Yiannouzis, 2010). This was highly controversial in the local community and in midwifery circles and led to a number of commentaries in relation to the decision (AIMS, 2010; Edwards and Davies, 2010; Walsh, 2010; Edwards, 2011).

Significant proportions of women attending the Albany Midwifery Practice were from BAME groups and/or single, both characteristics associated with poorer neonatal outcomes (Raleigh et al., 2010). This is in keeping with the local population which is highly ethnically diverse. In 2006, the ethnic profile of women using King's College Hospital maternity services included 42% who identified as Black African or Caribbean and only 43% who identified as White British (Demilew, 2007). This is more diverse than in greater London where from the most recent data, 60% of people residing in London are White British with 13% being Black/ African/ Caribbean/ Black British (13%) and 19% being Asian/Asian British Indian and 5% identifying as Mixed/ Multiple Ethnic Groups (Office for National Statistics, 2011).

It has been shown that women from BAME groups and single women are at higher risk of adverse outcomes during pregnancy and after. For example, these women are more likely to experience complications during pregnancy, an unplanned caesarean section, and having their baby cared for in a neonatal unit than those from the White British group (Raleigh et al., 2010). Babies of Black or Black British and Asian or Asian British ethnicity have also been shown to have the highest risk of extended perinatal mortality with rates of 9.8 and 8.8 per 1,000 total births respectively (Manktelow et al., 2015). These rates are considerably higher than the Albany rate of less than 2.0 per 1000 births in women from BAME groups (Table 8). In addition, in a UK survey, women in all minority ethnic groups had a poorer experience of maternity services than White women (Henderson et al., 2013) and expressed more worries about labour and birth (Redshaw and Heikkilä, 2011). While our study did not examine women's experiences, the fact that they had positive labour and birth outcomes suggests that they felt supported by the Albany Midwifery Practice. This is in keeping with a qualitative study where women from BAME backgrounds in an inner-city area identified that receiving caseload care enhanced the emotional social support they received from midwives, enabling them to feel safe, relaxed and able to confide about problems within a trusting relationship (Beake et al. 2013).

The preterm birth rate in our study was low (5.1%) with 94.8% of babies having an Apgar score of 8 or greater at 5 minutes and 6.2% admitted to a NNU for more than two days. There were 15 perinatal deaths over this period giving a perinatal mortality rate of 5.78 per 1000 total births. Two of the deaths were associated with significant congenital abnormalities and there were no intrapartum intrauterine deaths.

The perinatal mortality data for babies born through the Albany Midwifery Practice were lower than the rates for the United Kingdom over a similar period, where from 2000–2009, the perinatal mortality rate ranged from 7.5–8.5 per 1000 total births (Centre for Maternal and Child Enquiries (CMACE, 2011). The perinatal mortality rate in the Albany Midwifery Practice varied over the time period (1.8–7.7 per 1000 total births) although the absolute numbers were small (1–6 babies per 3–4 year time period). In addition, the rate of preterm births is lower than the national average. Between 2006–2010, the rate of preterm birth in the UK was 7–7.5% (Office of National Statistics, 2012); higher than the 5.1% rate in the Albany Midwifery Practice.

Our audit has shown that the Albany Midwifery Practice supported high rates of physiological births, a phenomenon described in a small study of midwifery caseload practice for similarly socially disadvantaged women (Rayment-Jones et al., 2015). In more than 12 years, almost 80% of women had spontaneous vaginal births and 16% had caesarean sections (12.2% emergency CS and 3.8% elective CS). The average caesarean section rate across England over that time ranged from 17–25% highlighting the lower rates in the Albany Midwifery Practice (Health and Social Care Information Centre, 2013).

The low incidence of birth assisted by forceps or ventouse (4.2%) may have been related to only 10% of women having an epidural in labour, given the identified increased risk of assisted vaginal birth associated with epidural analgesia (Anim-Somuah et al., 2005). Only 1.2% of women were given Pethidine and 15% used Entonox. Almost all women (95.5%) were supported by known midwives highlighting the value of midwifery continuity of care as a strategy to help women cope with pain as part of normal childbirth (Leap et al., 2010; Sanders and Lamb, 2014; Van der Gucht and Lewis, 2015; Sandall et al., 2016).

In this study, most women commenced labour spontaneously (80.5%)

and only 13.6% of labours involved induction, stimulation or augmentation of labour. The majority of women had no perineal trauma (62.2%); third degree tears were rare (0.7%), and the episiotomy rate was 3.8%. These results lend weight to evidence linking perineal trauma with episiotomy, induction of labour, epidural analgesia and assisted vaginal birth (Kudisha et al., 2008; Räisänen et al., 2010). There has been a suggestion that, where midwives reduce the number of episiotomies they perform, they tend to gain skill in preserving the woman's perineum intact (Begley, 2014). Data on the techniques used by Albany midwives were not collected; this raises the importance of recording such information so that it can be examined retrospectively in order to contribute to research in this area (Petrocnik and Marshall, 2015).

The majority (79%) of women who had a vaginal birth had a physiological third stage of labour. Of interest is that only 5.9% of women in this group had a blood loss of more than 500 ml. Similar outcomes have been recorded in large studies in New Zealand (Davis et al., 2012; Dixon et al., 2013). It has been suggested that midwives who are experienced in physiological third stage may have skills that protect women from excessive blood loss in normal labour (Jangsten et al., 2010; Begley et al., 2012; Begley, 2014).

Almost all (95.5%) women were attended in labour by their primary midwife or secondary midwife who they had got to know during pregnancy. Strong evidence has linked this relational continuity of care, often referred to as 'caseload midwifery,' to a reduction in the use of epidurals, episiotomies, instrumental births and pre-term births (Sandall et al., 2016). Caseload midwifery for women of any risk has also been associated with a reduction in elective CS, the use of pharmacological analgesia, induction of labour, and birth related blood loss, with an increase in the likelihood of continued breastfeeding after six weeks and six months and cost savings (Tracy et al., 2013).

The breastfeeding rates in women cared for by the Albany midwives were high: 91.5% initiated breastfeeding and 74.3% were still exclusively breastfeeding at 28 days (an additional 14.8% were mixed feeding). The promotion of breastfeeding is an important aspect of the public health role of midwives, with implications for addressing health inequalities and potential health gain (Department of Health, 2007a, 2010; Pokhrel et al., 2015).

The results of this audit add to the body of literature questioning the routine use of medico-technical interventions in labour (Begley, 2014; Johanson et al., 2002). They are of particular interest given that the women who accessed the Albany Midwifery Practice included those with pregnancies considered to be at all levels of obstetric, medical and social risk. Furthermore, the profile of the 2,568 women reflected that of the local population in Southwark, a high proportion being in groups considered to be most vulnerable in terms of socio-economic disadvantage and poor maternity outcomes (Department of Health, 2007b; Manktelow et al., 2015; Office for National Statistics 2016). In particular, women from BAME communities and single, unsupported mothers are more likely than White British women to experience complications, adverse outcomes, worry, and poor experiences of care during pregnancy and afterwards (Raleigh et al., 2010; Redshaw and Heikkilä, 2011; Henderson et al., 2013).

Midwifery continuity of carer can play an important role in addressing the needs of vulnerable women through the opportunity to build trusting relationships and access to safe, supportive services (McCourt and Pearce, 2000; Beake et al., 2001; Department of Health, 2010; Beake et al., 2013; ten Hoope-Bender, 2013; Manktelow et al., 2015). In previous studies, women who received care from Albany midwives have described a sense of calm and trust that this type of relational continuity of care engendered (Huber and Sandall, 2009). This gave them a chance to develop self-confidence as they approached the challenges of labour and new motherhood, including breastfeeding (Huber and Sandall, 2009; Leap et al., 2010).

One of the distinguishing features of the Albany Midwifery Practice model is access to, and support of, homebirth. The percentage of women who gave birth at home with the Albany midwives was 43.5%. Government documents in England have consistently promoted the idea that healthy women should be offered the choice of giving birth at home (Department of Health, 1993, 2004, 2007a); yet home birth has remained relatively uncommon over the years (below 3% in England). A large study comparing perinatal outcomes by planned place of birth (Birthplace in England Collaborative Group, 2011) supported a policy of offering women with low risk pregnancies a choice of birth settings, including birth at home (NICE, 2014). Despite such policy directives, the rates of homebirth remain static at 2.3% in 2012 and 2013 in England and Wales (Office for National Statistics, 2014).

The Albany midwives' practice included developing a positive culture around birth at home in the local community (Reed, 2015). The option to give birth at home remained open, including during labour, hence the changing proportion of women choosing this option as their pregnancies progressed. Caseload midwifery may allow more time and space for decision making to emerge fully, especially where home assessment in early labour allows for women to choose to stay at home or go to hospital, depending on how their labour is unfolding (Brintworth and Sandall, 2012).

Of the women who chose to give birth at home, 15.1% experienced transfer to hospital in labour (12.4% primiparous, 5.5% multiparous women). The implications of this are significant given the rates of transfer from home to an obstetric unit identified in the Birthplace in England (Birthplace in England Collaborative Group, 2011) study: 45% for primiparous women and 12% for multiparous women.

The proportion of women from BAME communities who gave birth at home with Albany midwives was lower than the proportion of White women. However, the fact that around one third of women from BAME groups gave birth at home is significant in light of the Birthplace in England Study (Birthplace in England Collaborative Group, 2011), which identified that women choosing to give birth at home were less likely to be in BAME groups.

We examined the data over 3–4 year time periods to see whether there were differences in demographic characteristics, practice and outcomes. The proportion of women identifying their ethnicity as White decreased significantly over time. It is interesting that over this time, the rate of waterbirth increased as did the proportion of women who planned a homebirth at 36 weeks. This could be explained by the growing confidence of the general population in the concept of waterbirth and the development of a local culture where birth at home with known midwives was seen as a normal and positive option for healthy women with uncomplicated pregnancies (Leap et al., 2010; Reed, 2015). An increase in the rate of homebirth is in contrast to practices in the majority of countries, where homebirth has decreased. For example, the home birth rate in the Netherlands is the highest in high income countries, although it has declined from 35 per cent of all births in 1997 to 2000 to 16 per cent of all births in 2013 despite strong evidence showing safety (Birthplace in England Collaborative Group, 2011; de Jonge et al., 2015). It is important to note that there were no significant changes in the rate of admission to a neonatal unit over these time periods.

Conclusion

An analysis of retrospective Albany Midwifery Practice statistics over 12.5 years has shown positive outcomes for women and babies in socially disadvantaged and BAME groups, including those with complex pregnancies and perceived risk factors. This study adds weight to a growing body of evidence linking relational midwifery continuity of carer with improved outcomes and policies identifying that all pregnant women should receive midwifery continuity of carer throughout the continuum of pregnancy, birth and new motherhood.

Appendix II

Campaign songs

(all lyrics by Rix Pyke)

To the tune of Let It Be:
   When you call the midwife – you are calling someone who can see –
   Birth's a natural process: Let it be
   If the midwife's frightened – or is bullied to conformity –
   The birth you want won't happen – can't you see?

   NMC NMC NMC NMC Midwives won't be bullied – let us be

   If protocols and guidelines take the place of flexibility
   Birth will be a nightmare – Let it be.
   If all of us are threatened by the fear of liability –
   This is not the answer – can't you see?
   NMC NMC etc

   Becky Reed's a midwife full of wisdom and integrity
   There is no case to answer NMC!
   If Becky is the iceberg there are hundreds more beneath the sea
   Midwives won't be bullied. Let us be
   Let us be let us be let us be let us be
   Speaking words of wisdom Let us be etc

To the tune of We Can Work It Out:
   Try to see it our way
   For the birth I want I need my midwife to be free
   If we do it your way
   We can lose the trust and then the fear is all you'll see
   We can work it out, we can work it out

   Think of what I'm saying
   See our midwives frightened to do what they know is right
   Think of what you're doing

Turning all our midwives into scapegoats overnight
We can work it out we can work it out

Chorus: Birth is long or short it's all the same –
it need not be frightening my friend
Midwives walk the talk and won't be blamed –
and so we'll tell you once again my friends :
Try to see it our way etc..

To the tune of Show me the way to go home:
Show me the way to have a home birth
I'm tired of this hospital bed
I got to know my midwife 'bout an hour ago
And now another one's here instead.
I wish I was at home
Feeling safe and calm and warm
Not lying here with strangers in this clinical room
Oh show me the way to have a home birth.

Show me the way to have a home birth
Let me tell you what I mean
Not feeling like I've only got an hour to go
Til they have to intervene.
I won't be told to push
Or bossed or scared or rushed
I'll take however long it takes
To finish the job
Oh show me the way to have a home birth!

To the tune of Robin Hood, Robin Hood riding thru the glen:
NMC NMC this is not the end
NMC NMC we'll drive you round the bend
Here we will wait 'til you exonerate
Becky Reed Becky Reed Becky Reed

To the tune of It's a long way to Tipperary:
It is no way to have a baby
On a conveyor belt
It is no way to have a baby

If only fear and pain is felt
How long's a *normal* labour?
How long's a piece of string!?
It is just no way to have a baby
With a clock tick-tocking.

It is no way to have a baby
Without people you know
It is no way to have a baby
Feeling rushed – not safe and slow
Goodbye legs in stirrups
Farewell facing the wall
It is just no way to have a baby
It's not 'one size fits all!'

To the tune of Roll Out the Barrel:
    Roll out the model
    The Albany model is best
    Roll out the model
    We want it North, South, East and West.
    Roll out the model
    It's what women want over here
    So hurry and roll out the model
    With continuity of care!
     Roll out the model
    The Albany model is fine
    Roll out the model
    They know that a labour takes time
    Roll out the model
    For birthing is not a disease
    So hurry and roll out the model
    And let us all have Albanys.

To the tune of of Swing Low, Sweet Chariot:
    Sink low and close the practice
    Now's the time to say what's been done
    Sink low and close the practice

Now's the time to say what's been done

You go down to Peckham and what do you see?
Now's the time to say what's been done
A whole load of people as angry as can be
Now's the time to say what's been done

Sink low etc...

They closed down the practice
And sullied their name
Now's the time to say what's been done
They massaged statistics in order to blame
Now's the time to say what's been done

Sink low etc...

All of King's Healthcare should quiver in shame
Now's the time to say what's been done

Our midwives are innocent so now clear their name
Now's the time to say what's been done

Sink low etc...

The Albany midwives have kindled a spark
Now's the time to say what's been done
A beacon of hope it has shone in the dark
Now's the time to say what's been done
Sink low etc.

To the tune of The Lion Sleeps Tonight:
    Pt 1: The Albany the Albany
    The Albany the Albany
    The Albany the Albany
    The Albany the Albany (repeat ad. naus)

    Pt 2: Down in Peckham, way down in Peckham
    The Albany shone bright
    Down in Peckham, way down in Peckham
    The Albany shone bright... (*repeat etc...*)

    Pt 3: Ah woah! Now is the time to clear their name.
    Ah woah! Now is the time to clear their name.... (*repeat etc...*)

Albany carols – written for the event in Whitehall (all lyrics Rix Pyke)

To the tune of Oh come all ye faithful:
    Oh come all ye pregnant
    Tell us all what matters
    Oh come ye oh come ye
    And tell us the truth:

    We want it loving, caring, calm and private
    We don't want strangers watching
    We want to know who's catching
    We want our babies latching on

    With continuity!
    You need to hear us
    Birth is not an illness
    We want it where we want

    And on our own terms:
    We want it loving, caring, calm and private
    We don't want strangers watching
    We want to know who's catching
    We want our babies latching on
    With continuity.

To the tune of Away in a manger:
    Give birth with a stranger – why, whatever for?
    It's a time when you need to feel safe and secure.
    We don't want to be hurried or hustled or scared

    We want to be quietly and calmly prepared.
    Our wonderful midwives have done this so well
    So why would we choose to give birth in a hell?
    The Albany Practice has ignited a spark
    They've long been a beacon which shines in the dark.

To the tune of We three kings:
    We see King's is going too far
    Closing down our shining bright star
    Is women choosing Too confusing?

Let us show you who we are!

Chorus: Ooohh star of wonder star of light
The Albany will see you right
Is women choosing too confusing
Let us all keep up the fight!

Black and white and from far and near
We all want to birth without fear
And so the fact is
Our Albany Practice
Gives continuity of care!

Chorus: Ooohh star of wonder star of light
The Albany will see you right
Is women choosing too confusing
Let us all keep up the fight!

Harken ye in all your white coats
From old Land's End to John o'Groats
The Albany shines
In our hearts and minds
A beacon of sense and love and hope!

Chorus: Ooohh star of wonder star of light
The Albany will see you right
Is women choosing too confusing
Let us all keep up the fight!

List of abbreviations

AAG	Albany Action Group
AIMS	Association for Improvements in the Maternity Services
AMAG	Albany Model Advisory Group
AMP	Albany Midwifery Practice
ARM	Association of Radical Midwives
CE/CEO	Chief Executive
CEMACH	Confidential Enquiry into Maternal and Child Health
CHRE	Council for Healthcare Regulatory Excellence
CMACE	Centre for Maternal and Child Enquiries
CQC	Care Quality Commission
FoI	Freedom of Information
GP	General Practitioner
HIE	Hypoxic Ischaemic Encephalopathy
JFMBR	Justice for Midwife Becky Reed
KCH	King's College Hospital
LSA	Local Supervising Authority
LSAMO	Local Supervising Authority Midwifery Officer
MP	Member of Parliament
MSLC	Maternity Services Liaison Committee
NCT	National Childbirth Trust
NE	Neonatal Encephalopathy
NHS	National Health Service
NICE	National Institute for Health and Care Excellence
NMC	Nursing and Midwifery Council
NPEU	National Perinatal Epidemiology Unit
PCT	Primary Care Trust
RCM	Royal College of Midwives
SCBU	Special Care Baby Unit
SELMGP	South East London Midwifery Group Practice
SHA	Strategic Health Authority

Acknowledgements

Piecing together this story has been a monumental and challenging task. We could not have done it without the support and encouragement of so many people. We would like to say a huge thank you to the following:

The Albany midwives at the time of the closure – Mary Ardill, Fran Chambers, Danielle Clover (Nixon), Sophie Cunningham (Whitecross), Natalie Doherty, Melissa Earle, Zoe Lench, Nicky O'Brien (Gibbs), Zoe Vowles.

All those who agreed to be interviewed for the book.

All those who have written an individual contribution to the book.

The Albany Mums, especially Emma Beamish.

The organisations that supported the Albany at the time of the closure – Association for Improvements in the Maternity Services (AIMS), the NCT (formerly National Childbirth Trust), Association of Radical Midwives.

The members of the Save The Albany/Albany Action Group campaign.

The members of AMAG (Albany Model Advisory Group).

Pauline Armstrong (Albany practice manager) for her extraordinary work during the time of the closure.

Beverley Beech for her tireless activism during the campaign.

Sarah Davies for being with us every step of the way, for being Becky's 'right-hand woman' and for co-writing the chapter about Becky's investigation.

Vicky Garner for her enthusiasm and expertise in setting up and managing the Justice for Midwife Becky Reed Facebook page.

Caroline Homer, Nicky Leap and Jane Sandall for the vital Albany Midwifery Practice outcomes paper.

Mavis Kirkham for the Foreword, and for her belief in the campaign and her insightful contributions.

Janet Lightfoot for her prompt and accurate transcriptions of our interviews.

Alison Macfarlane for her professional untangling of the statistics in the story.

Jackie Moulla for her encouragement and friendship as Becky's midwifery supervisor.

Jo Murphy-Lawless for her wisdom and acuity during the campaign and Becky's investigation.

Elizabeth Prochaska for her invaluable personal and professional support for Becky.

Rix Pyke for writing the witty and inspirational lyrics for the campaign songs.

Sara Wickham for her generous and knowledgeable support during the writing of the book.

Luke Zander for his decades-long unwavering commitment to the Albany model of care.

All those who read and commented on the first draft of the book – Mary Ardill, Pauline Armstrong, Andy Beckingham, Clare Bee, Gill Boden, Fran Chambers, Danielle Clover, Sophie Cunningham, Sarah Davies, Natalie Doherty, Zoe Lench, Laura Lightfoot, Tim Lightfoot, Nicky Macphail, Nicky O'Brien, Cath Pilley, Adrian Reed, Jenny Rutt, Cat Scott, Zoe Vowles, Cathy Walton and Sara Wickham.

Martin Wagner and Susan Last at Pinter & Martin for their commitment to this book, and for their limitless patience during the writing of it.

And finally... our husbands Adrian and Peter, who were by our sides when we had our first babies in 1976, have supported our work over the decades, and believed strongly in the importance of telling this story.

About the authors

Becky Reed

For almost all my adult life I have been passionate about the politics of maternity. Pregnant for the first time in 1976, I contacted the NCT looking for good pregnancy care, and got it from a wonderful GP, Charles Mansfield, who saw me throughout my pregnancy and came to my birth. Charles offered me relational continuity, and I am eternally grateful to him for opening my eyes to its importance. My husband Adrian and I went to antenatal classes with Caroline Flint, who taught us about choice and autonomy and our rights as 'users' in the increasingly interventionist world of birth. I was shocked to discover the truths about expected practices at the time (for example lying flat in labour and an almost 100% episiotomy rate), and fought to give birth as normally as possible, even though my feet were 'too small' and my baby chose to stay inside until nearly 43 weeks.

After Laura's birth I was energised and motivated. I became the booking secretary for the local branch of the NCT, had a second baby at home in 1978, and then was persuaded by Caroline to train as an antenatal teacher. I taught NCT classes for 15 years, during which time I had two more babies at home, and enjoyed being with my children in that now very rare role of full-time mother. I was one of a group of local women who trained as NCT teachers together; we became close friends, had babies together, formed a 'Women's Group' together, and supported each other through those often difficult early years of parenting.

Listening to the experiences of the couples who came to my classes I realised that there was work to be done, and that if I was going to change the (maternity) world I needed to get on to the front line and train as a midwife. So with four young children, and supported by my husband Adrian and all those wonderful friends, I embarked on midwifery training. I found the impersonal, fragmented care in the hospital difficult and upsetting, and I cried most days. At the end of the course my tutor begged me to 'stay and help us to change things from the inside', but I knew I couldn't work in the system a moment longer. At that time there was no option to work in the NHS in the way I believed in, and even those planning to be community midwives had to spend two years in the hospital to 'consolidate' their learning. I wanted nothing less than to consolidate the practices that I had observed and struggled with as a student, so I left, feeling the need to reconnect with my family, see my youngest child into school, and think carefully about what to do next.

I had found a new community in the Association of Radical Midwives (ARM), and had been attending meetings locally for a few years. Within a few months I felt confident enough to set up as an independent midwife, and worked in this way for a few wonderfully rewarding years, always hoping that the opportunity would arise to set up a similar way of working within the NHS.

That opportunity came in the early nineties with the publication of the government document *Changing Childbirth*. To those of us supporting each other as independent midwives in south-east London this was what we had been working towards. The time was right and we were able to begin to realise our dream of offering continuity of carer within the NHS. (For more about this see Chapter 2.) I had been learning from women for the previous few years about how birth really works and what matters to them, and my faith in the maternity system was all but destroyed. But here was the chance to change that world, to offer a new possibility and fresh hope. We grabbed that chance with both hands.

The story of what happened over the next 15 years is here in this book. I will always be grateful that I became a midwife when I did, and was able to work as a real midwife for so long. And I will always be so sad that my dream for the future of maternity care in the UK has yet to be realised.

Following my protracted and painful NMC investigation, I realised that, although the outcome was that there was no case to answer, I was battered and bruised and my Practice was closed. My barrister friend Elizabeth asked me to be her midwife, which was the best vindication I could have wished for, and Anton's beautiful birth in February 2014 was my last as an 'official' midwife. I deregistered as a midwife the following spring. Since then I have worked as an occasional doula, run a weekly postnatal group, done some writing and speaking, and been an active grandmother to my 12 grandchildren! And in 2016 my first book was published: *Birth in Focus,* a collection of birth stories in words and photos from my time as a midwife in Peckham.

It has taken me a long time to be able to write this book. The emotions are raw and profound, and the sense of injustice endures. I always knew that I wouldn't be able to write the story on my own, and the fact that Nadine agreed to co-author the book is what has made it possible. She has brought to it an unparalleled commitment, an unwavering belief in its importance, huge professionalism, and an enormous amount of good humour. I cannot thank her enough.

Nadine Edwards

Priviliged to now be a mother of three and a grandmother of five, I was unwittingly launched into the politics of maternity care when I was first pregnant in 1976. As a young and naive (at least in the field of birth) pregnant woman in the Scottish Borders, I gaily went to see my GP to plan a home birth. I was puzzled and taken aback when my GP told me that if I persisted with this idea I would be struck off his list. I was told horror stories about home births so I searched for any research about safety in birth. Margaret Whyte of the Society to Support Home Confinements sent me useful information about Marjorie Tew's work and about my rights. I could see nothing to suggest that I was committing a dangerous or foolish act and still believed that I could best protect my baby from the potential harms of unnecessary interventions by having as straightforward a birth as possible at home. Feminism, human rights, birth politics, power differentials and more came starkly together. My passion was ignited: I understood that while pregnant women had rights, those rights were being undermined. Surely women and babies deserved better, surely an injustice was being done in the name of safety that seemed from my limited understanding to be flawed. After leaving my GP's surgery that day I devoted myself to supporting women to navigate the politics and practices of birth. I started by helping a few women who wanted to avoid unnecessary interventions during a time when these were routinely carried out. The Association for Improvements in the Maternity Services (AIMS) invited me to join in 1980 and I worked voluntarily for the organisation for 35 years. During this time I wrote about birth, was involved in research and completed a PhD on women's experiences of birth. I remain grounded in and hugely value my work with women through the pregnancy and postnatal groups that I set up in my own home in 1985. These eventually led to a local charity, the Pregnancy and Parents Centre, being established in Edinburgh. It is the women's stories, insights and experiences that inspire me to seek justice, love, care and nurturing in the maternity services that are all too often indifferent, even abusive.

In the course of this work, I learned of the plight of the Albany Midwives in the late summer of 2009. For me, the Albany Midwifery Practice was a stunning beacon of what midwifery can mean for families and communities – how midwives can reduce the harmful impacts of inequalities by providing love and care at times of vulnerability. It gave me hope where often there seemed little to be hopeful about in maternity services. It was not only the phenomenally good outcomes of the Practice that inspired me, but also the way the midwives worked with their community. I had a close affinity with their deeply political understanding of health and inequalities, promoting and respecting women's agency, developing trusting, safe relationships with women and families who had often experienced a profound lack of safety, working with the whole community and supporting women to develop their own networks of support that would last a lifetime rather than the few months that the midwives could be involved in their lives. The midwives' care, their belief in the women and their focus on nurturing the women's belief in themselves and their abilities to be pregnant, birth their babies and be capable mothers was outstanding. The value of this in a disparate, challenged community, to my mind, was something that most maternity services (with some shining exceptions) were nowhere near achieving and are currently further away from than ever. When I discovered that the Albany Midwifery Practice was under threat I was shocked beyond belief. We had already lost many small midwifery services that had been keeping alive a skilled, individualised, caring approach in an increasingly technological, often dehumanised obstetric service delivered in large centralised units. Losing the Albany seemed to be the death knell of midwifery services – if it fell, we all fell. I could not stand by and do nothing.

The campaigns were challenging and exhausting but at the same time it was a privilege to work with the Albany Mums who did so much, the Albany midwives, the activists, the researchers, midwives and other practitioners. It has also been an honour to work with Becky in the crafting of this story that so needed to be told. My appreciation of her during the campaigns to keep the Albany Midwifery Practice alive and during the writing of this book over too many years to mention has deepened exponentially. To write with a colleague, friend and fellow activist of such moral courage, insight and ethical standing is an invaluable honour. It is due to her meticulous record-keeping that it has been possible to tell the story in such detail and with the confidence that it accurately reflects events as they unfolded. The unbearable distress of seeing the Albany Midwifery Practice dismantled and the trauma of Becky's case has been eased by working together on this venture to bring a story of a profound injustice to light.

My work has been made possible by my family's consistent understanding of the importance of childbirth. The support that they have given me is a gift without which I could not have worked in the way that I have. Many remarkable women, birth activists, midwives, researchers and doctors have helped me to learn about the complex politics of midwifery and birth. They have taught me to question, write and act in ways I would not have otherwise thought possible.

Index